101 AMAZING USES for TURMERIC

FAMILIUS

FOR MY PARKLAND COMMUNITY
#MSDSTRONG

Published by Familius LLC, www.familius.com

Familius books are available at special discounts for bulk purchases, whether for sales promotions or for family or corporate use. For more information, contact Familius Sales at 559-876-2170 or email orders@familius.com.

DISCLAIMER: The material in this book is for informational purposes only. It is not intended to be a substitute for professional medical advice, diagnosis, or treatment. Always seek the advice of your physician or other qualified healthcare provider with any questions you may have regarding a medical condition or treatment. Never disregard professional medical advice or delay in seeking it because of something you have read in this book.

Library of Congress Cataloging-in-Publication Data
2018936021

Print ISBN 9781945547928
Ebook ISBN 9781641700573

Printed in the United States of America

Edited by Leah Welker
Cover design by David Miles
Book design by Brooke Jorden and Caroline Larsen

10 9 8 7 6 5 4 3 2 1
First Edition

101 AMAZING USES for TURMERIC

REDUCE JOINT PAIN, SOOTHE YOUR STOMACH, MAKE A DELICIOUS DINNER, AND 98 MORE!

Susan Branson

CONTENTS

CHAPTER 2: ATTAIN PHYSICAL AND MENTAL WELLNESS | 65

CHAPTER 3: ACCENTUATE BEAUTY | 99

CHAPTER 4: APPLY IN ARTS AND CRAFTS | 119

NOTES | 129

INTRODUCTION

TURMERIC, THE ROOT OF MANY USES

Most people buy turmeric as a deep yellow powder in the spice aisle. It may be surprising to see turmeric whole, in its rhizome form.

The rhizome is actually the horizontal, underground stem of the plant. From this, the upright stem containing the leaves and flowers rises about a meter above the surface. Below the ground, roots branch off the rhizome to reach down into the earth. Often, the rhizome is referred to as a root, so when you see the term *turmeric root*, it actually refers to the rhizome.

Turmeric looks very similar to ginger and, in fact, is part of the ginger family. The main rhizome tends to grow up to three inches long and an inch in diameter, with smaller rhizomes branching off in all directions. The rhizomes are tuberous, segmented, and rough in appearance. The outside of the turmeric rhizome is a yellowish-brown color, and the inside is orange, similar to that of a carrot.

The rhizomes are harvested, boiled for roughly forty minutes, dried in ovens, and then ground into the familiar yellowish-orange powder. Most often used as a spice in Indian and Southeast Asian dishes and as one of the main spices in curry, turmeric has a sweet yet slightly bitter flavor that pairs well with coconut, chilies, beef, poultry, seafood, and other spices like pepper, cumin, ginger, and nutmeg, among others. Turmeric is used equally for its flavor and its color. Depending on the amount used, it will turn a dish any shade between soft butter-yellow to strong marigold. Its suitability as a dye has encouraged the food, textile, and beauty industries to use turmeric to color food, cloth, and cosmetic products.

The yellow color of turmeric comes from one of its main constituents, a polyphenol called curcumin, comprising about 6 percent of the rhizome. Over the last few decades, the medical community began taking notice of turmeric, and now thousands of studies have identified turmeric and curcumin as having antioxidant, anti-inflammatory, antimicrobial, anticancer, and hypoglycemic properties. These have the potential for far-reaching applications, and we have been hearing more and more about the beneficial healing effects of turmeric on conditions that are both chronic and acute, common and rare, minor and serious.

TURMERIC'S ENDURING HISTORY

Turmeric has been used for over four thousand years, with its origins lying in Southeast Asia or India. First used as a spice in food and in religious ceremonies, it soon became recognized and revered for its holistic healing properties in Ayurvedic and Unani traditional medical practices in these regions. They used turmeric to calm swelling, heal wounds, alleviate gas, eliminate worms, improve digestion, and treat respiratory and liver disorders. Even a written prescription for the use of turmeric to relieve the ill effects of poisoned food is recorded in Suśruta's *Compendium*, an ancient Indian text on medicine and surgery.

As turmeric's reputation rose, its demand spread, and soon this spice was found all over Asia, Africa, and Europe. In his legendary travels, Marco Polo spoke of discovering a wonderfully colorful root, similar in quality to saffron. He was referring to the beautiful orange color of turmeric. No doubt turmeric's label as "Indian saffron" is partly attributable to Polo's comment. Subsequently, turmeric eclipsed saffron's popularity as a dye for food and clothing. This was because turmeric acted as a superior dye to saffron and was much less expensive.

Today, India is still the largest producer, consumer, and exporter of turmeric. The average person there consumes anywhere from 100 to 200 milligrams per day,[1] much more than the average North American. The tradition of using turmeric in religious ceremonies has endured in some parts of Indian culture. Brides and grooms apply turmeric paste to their faces and bodies before the wedding as part of a purification ritual and to calm the nerves. In other regions, a groom ties a turmeric-dyed yellow string around his bride's neck as a symbol of entering a sacred and successful marriage and to ensure fertility.

In North America, turmeric is mainly used as a spice in food but also as a dye. However, the medicinal properties of turmeric have risen in popularity. In the early 18th century, Vogel and Pelletier isolated curcumin from the rhizomes of turmeric, and following scientists began to discover the amazing array of properties curcumin has. In 1937, Oppenheimer published the first article on the effects of curcumin on human disease, specifically inflammation of the gallbladder.[2] Since that time, numerous research, including clinical trials, have identified the vastly important and far-reaching potential turmeric has in human health.

THE DIFFERENT WAYS TO USE TURMERIC

Turmeric can be found as a powder, as a fresh root (rhizome), or even in pickled form. It can also be taken as a supplement. Ground turmeric is made by peeling, boiling, drying, then grinding the roots. Most of us go directly to the baking aisle in the grocery store and pick up a small jar of the dry, ground spice. It's easy to use, and it stores up to two years. It tends to start losing potency after about six months, though. Shelf life can be prolonged by keeping the spice in a jar with a tight-fitting lid and placing it in a cool, dark cupboard. Sunlight and heat will speed degradation. Sometimes the root is dried and sold whole, but you may have to look in specialty stores or Asian markets to find this form. It is interesting to note that the process of boiling and roasting fresh turmeric to make the dry rhizome and powder increases its antioxidant potency.[3, 4]

Fresh turmeric roots can be peeled and either chopped into small pieces or grated with a Microplane and used in a variety of dishes. Raw turmeric can be juiced or added to smoothies. Cooking with turmeric adds an abundance of healthful benefits, a mildly bitter or pungent flavor, and a beautiful yellow color. When selecting fresh turmeric, choose one that is firm and smooth, without wrinkles. Be careful to avoid any with mold. The root can be wrapped in paper towel, sealed in a plastic bag, and stored in the refrigerator for up to two weeks. If freezing, it can be stored for up to six months or longer. Note that freezing turmeric will soften the consistency, but the flavor should remain strong. As a general rule of thumb, when cooking with turmeric, 1 inch of fresh turmeric equates to about 1 teaspoon of ground turmeric.

Pickled turmeric is made by peeling the root and slicing it into bite-sized pieces. This will stain the hands, so kitchen gloves are recommended. The turmeric pieces are placed in a glass jar with lemon juice and apple cider vinegar. The jar is sealed and refrigerated for about a week before being ready. It should be consumed over the next three months.

Turmeric supplements are offered as a method of obtaining the medicinal benefits of turmeric in a convenient package. They come as tablets or capsules that contain either turmeric root powder or concentrated curcumin extracted from the root. Because most of the health benefits come from curcumin, it is recommended that those looking for supplements choose one that has curcumin quantities standardized to a high percentage.

When taking turmeric for health purposes, it is important to note that the bioavailability (the proportion used by the body) of curcumin is very low. Only small amounts are absorbed into the bloodstream. Adding piperine, found in black pepper, to curcumin increases bioavailability by 2000 percent.[5] Alternatively, combining turmeric with a fat, such as coconut oil, also increases bioavailability. Curcumin binds to the fat and is then carried through the intestinal wall and into the bloodstream, where it becomes available for use in the body.

HOW MUCH SHOULD I USE?

Studies on the beneficial effects of turmeric have used anywhere from 0.5 grams to 6 grams per day of whole turmeric powder. Other studies have used curcumin extracted from turmeric, in amounts ranging from 1 gram to 4 grams per day. Quantities were given for up to nine months of daily use and appeared to be well tolerated, safe, and effective at their intended therapeutic purpose. One study set out to find the maximum tolerable dosage of curcumin and gave subjects escalating dosages to a maximum of 12 grams. All doses were found to be safe in human subjects.[6] It should be noted that several participants did experience some minor side effects and that this study only tested a single dose, not consecutive daily dosages as would be used to improve health conditions. For such benefits, the University of Maryland Medical Center recommends taking between 1 and 3 grams of turmeric powder per day. This would equate to about 1/3 to 1 teaspoon per day. There are not specific recommendations for children, but dosage can be determined by weight. As a guideline, if a child is about 50 pounds, use 1/3 the recommended amount for adults.

IS TAKING TURMERIC SAFE?

When taken at the recommended dosages, both turmeric and curcumin are generally recognized as safe by the FDA. High doses consumed orally may cause diarrhea, nausea, or upset stomach. As with any substance, allergies can occur, and some people have reported a mild, itchy rash after topical use. Oral consumption may negatively impact health if conditions involving the gallbladder, gastroesophageal reflux, and iron deficiency exist. Caution should also be taken to avoid turmeric before surgery or in cases of bleeding disorders. It is known to slow blood clotting. Large amounts can stimulate the uterus, so pregnant women need to be extra vigilant in keeping track of their consumption.

Make sure to check with your doctor before consuming turmeric if you take medication. Turmeric can slow down the metabolism of certain drugs and increase their side effects. It can work synergistically with drugs, too, and overproduce results. Taking diabetes drugs in combination with turmeric can cause blood sugar levels to dip too low. Diabetics also need to be aware that taking turmeric with other blood sugar–lowering herbs like devil's claw, garlic, and ginseng may also cause this effect.

CHAPTER 1

ALLEVIATE ILLNESS AND INFECTION

1. ACQUIRED IMMUNO-DEFICIENCY SYNDROME (AIDS)

HIV, or human immunodeficiency virus, is a sexually transmitted disease that can be spread through bodily fluids from an infected person to another person or from mother to child during pregnancy, birth, or breastfeeding. HIV attacks the body's immune system and destroys cells the body uses to fight off infections and disease. Opportunistic infections and cancers can develop and spread unabated. There are three stages of the disease. The first stage can last for several weeks, and those infected may experience fever, headache, sore throat, and muscle pain. The second stage often has no symptoms, and if antiretroviral medications are taken, the progression can be slowed for decades. Without treatment, the immune system gets badly damaged, and within a decade, the disease progresses to stage three, known as AIDS. The body is susceptible to many infections at this stage, and survival time dramatically decreases. Once HIV is detected, treatment with a combination of anti-HIV drugs should begin to keep viral levels low. Unfortunately, there is no cure for HIV.

Curcumin from turmeric has shown promise as an antiretroviral compound that can act at different stages of the HIV life cycle and slow its progression in the body. It does this by inhibiting the virus from inserting its DNA into human genetic material[7] and by preventing HIV protease (an enzyme that breaks proteins apart) from making more viruses.[8] Evidence for the inhibition of other viral enzymes essential to HIV replication and spread have also been identified.[9, 10] Curcumin shows promise as an agent in the development of antiviral drugs to be used for slowing down or halting the advancement of HIV and AIDS.

2. ALLERGIES

They can strike in spring when pollen fills the air, at a friend's house when their cute ginger kitten rubs against your leg, or after eating the most satisfying lunch at the local popular seafood restaurant. Allergic reactions can cause minor irritations that result in a stuffy nose, watery eyes, or mild headache or potentially be so severe as to threaten life. They happen when the immune system reacts to a substance, whether it's swirling through in the air, absorbed through the skin, or eaten for lunch. While these substances don't cause a problem for most people, the immune system of someone with an allergy sees the trigger substance as an unwelcome invader and launches an attack against it. Specific antibodies are produced for each allergen that identify it as harmful to the body. Every time a person comes in contact with that allergen, the allergic response is activated.

There is no cure for allergies, but there are many over-the-counter and prescription drugs available to help ease symptoms. Among these are antihistamines, decongestants, and corticosteroids. They can cause drowsiness, high blood pressure, insomnia, irritability, restricted urine flow, muscle weakness, fluid retention, and weight gain—and these are just some of the side effects. This seems like trading one set of symptoms for another.

Turmeric has traditionally been used to treat allergies. In a food allergy study using mice, turmeric, but not curcumin, significantly lowered allergy symptoms as evidenced by a decrease in rectal temperature and anaphylactic response. Curcumin only showed a weak response, indicating that other compounds in turmeric are responsible for its effect.[11] Curcumin is capable of lowering the allergic response to environmental allergens, however. In allergic asthmatics exposed to dust mites, curcumin inhibited the formation of cytokines, chemicals that play a role in the production of antibodies and airway inflammation.[12] In patients with hay fever that were given either placebo or oral curcumin for 2 months, curcumin alleviated runny nose, sneezing, and nasal congestion.[13] It appears as though curcumin is very effective in reducing the symptoms of environmental allergies, while turmeric is more effective for food allergies.

3. ALZHEIMER'S

Alzheimer's disease—a form of dementia—is a progressive brain disorder that is irreversible. It can begin with memory loss and result in wandering and getting lost, repeating questions, and some personality and behavioral changes. As it progresses, memory loss and confusion grow worse, and people may have trouble recognizing friends and family, carrying out multi-step tasks, or coping with new situations. In the late stage, brain tissue shrinks significantly, and communication becomes difficult. Alzheimer's patients become completely dependent on others for care and often become bedridden. In most people with Alzheimer's, symptoms begin in their mid-sixties, although complex brain changes can begin years earlier. Current treatment approaches encourage patients to focus on mental function and manage behavioral symptoms. Several medications have been approved by the US FDA for the treatment of these symptoms.

The administration of curcumin to patients in a six-month clinical pilot study found increased levels of serum Aβ peptides in the brains compared to those in the placebo group that did not receive any curcumin.[14] The Aβ peptide consists of the amino acids that make up a plaque in the brains of Alzheimer's patients; the plaque causes nerve cell death and the degeneration of brain function. This evidence suggests that curcumin is able to collect Aβ deposits in the brain and release them into the blood, where they can be sent for disposal. Removing the deposits responsible for the symptoms of Alzheimer's would provide a safe way to prevent or even reverse this disease.

4. ASTHMA

Asthma is a chronic condition in which the airways leading to the lungs are inflamed. When exposed to triggers (chemicals or situations that impact the body), the airways swell and produce extra mucus. The passageway for air narrows, and breathing becomes more difficult. Symptoms include coughing, shortness of breath, wheezing, and chest pain. Anyone can develop asthma, although some are genetically predisposed to it. Triggers can be allergens, both environmental and food, or other substances like smoke, pollution, or changes in the weather. Learning what your specific triggers are goes a long way toward asthma management. Doctors often prescribe controller medications like corticosteroids and long-acting beta agonists and sometimes leukotriene modifiers to help manage the condition. Short-acting beta agonists are pre-scribed to quickly relieve symptoms by relaxing and opening the airways.

Because of the increasing and alarming rise of asthma in chil-dren and adults, it is more important than ever to find ways to manage this condition without the overuse of controller medica-tions. Curcumin from turmeric is showing promise as a potential anti-asthmatic treatment. Guinea pigs were sensitized to develop asthma symptoms. When treated with curcumin during the sen-sitization phase, the usual hyper-reactive response to histamine was significantly reduced. Histamine is a compound that is part of the body's immune system and is designed to rid the body of allergens. When triggered, it induces inflammation at the site of the reaction—in this case, the lungs. In another group of guinea pigs, curcumin was administered after airway inflammation and constriction. A significant reduction in swelling was noted.[15] Consuming turmeric on a daily basis may be an effective means of helping to control the symptoms of asthma.

5. ATHEROSCLEROSIS

When plaque builds up inside the arteries, atherosclerosis results. This plaque is comprised of cholesterol, fat, calcium, cellular waste products, and fibrin, a protein involved in blood clotting. Over time, the plaque builds up on the artery wall and hardens. The artery opening narrows, and the flow of oxygen-rich blood to the body is reduced. Arteries to the heart, brain, arms, legs, kidneys or pelvis may be involved. If a piece of the plaque breaks off and is carried to another part of the body, it can get stuck in a smaller artery and cut off blood flow to that part of the body. Sometimes blood clots form on the surface of plaque and block the artery entirely at the site of the plaque. If the blockage is to the heart, a heart attack will result. If it's to the head, a stroke occurs.

Atherosclerosis can begin in childhood but most often presents itself later in life. Smoking, a sedentary lifestyle, high blood pressure, poor diet, and genetics are all risk factors that can lead to its development. Changes in lifestyle and ongoing medical care are often required to minimize damage and manage this disease.

The oxidation of low density lipoprotein cholesterol (LDL) contributes to the development of atherosclerosis. A turmeric extract was found to decrease the susceptibility of LDL to oxidation in rabbits and protect them from the consequences inherent in the progression of the disease.[16] Another animal study mixed a low dose of curcumin from turmeric into a Western diet that was fed to mice over a four-month period. It was established that curcumin inhibited the development of plaque on their artery walls.[17] From these results, turmeric appears to be very beneficial in preventing plaque formation in arterial walls and can slow or halt the progression of this potentially deadly disease.

HEALTH

WELLNESS

BEAUTY

CRAFTS

6. BREAST CANCER

Breast cancer starts when cells of the breast begin to grow out of control and form a tumor. Tumors are cancerous if they grow and spread into other areas of the body. The condition is much more common in women, but men can get breast cancer, too. Early detection can be made through mammograms before symptoms begin. If not detected early, breast cancer can cause bloody discharge from the nipple or changes in the shape or texture of the breast or nipple. It can also be felt as a lump. Treatment may involve radiation, chemotherapy, or surgery.

This is the most common cancer among women, so finding new and effective therapies is critical to help increase survival rates. Harnessing the power of natural products, like curcumin in turmeric, can provide a safe and effective means of fighting breast cancer. The action of curcumin on human breast cancer cells was investigated in a recent study. Curcumin was toxic to the breast cancer cells and induced their death in both a time- and dose-dependent manner.[18] Whether used alone as a daily supplement for preventative purposes or in combination with other therapies to combat breast cancer, curcumin has proven to be beneficial in the fight against this cancer.

7. BRONCHITIS

Bronchitis is a respiratory disease characterized by the inflammation of the lining of the bronchial airways of the lungs. Acute bronchitis can result from a cold or other respiratory infection causing the mucus membranes to swell and air pathways to narrow. Chronic bronchitis is more severe and is a constant inflammation of the lining of the bronchial tubes, most often caused by smoking. People with bronchitis have coughing spells and often cough up mucus. Chest pain, fever, chills, and fatigue are other symptoms. Acute bronchitis often goes away on its own after a short time, while chronic bronchitis persists and often requires cough medicine, asthma inhalers, or antibiotics if a bacterial infection is suspected.

In adults and healthy, older children, the respiratory syncytial virus causes symptoms of a mild cold. In babies and young children, however, it is the major cause of bronchitis. Respiratory distress can be alarming for parents and frightening for children. Curcumin has been found to prevent the respiratory syncytial virus from replicating and spreading in human nasal epithelial cells, the protective outermost layer of cells inside the nose. No toxicity to the cells was observed.[19] Curcumin can be used to treat bronchitis in children, although the introduction of any spices to infants younger than eight months is not recommended. Turmeric milk is an effective way to have the child consume curcumin.

HOT TURMERIC MILK FOR CHILDREN

1/8 inch fresh turmeric root, peeled
1/8 inch fresh ginger root, peeled
1 tablespoon raw honey
pinch of black pepper
pinch of cinnamon (optional)
1 cup milk

1. Combine all ingredients in a food processor or blender until the roots have been puréed. Pour into a saucepan and heat.
2. For adult consumption, increase the amounts of turmeric and ginger to 1/2 inch each.

8. CANDIDIASIS

Candidiasis is a fungal infection caused by the yeast-like *Candida* fungus. There are over twenty species of *Candida* that can infect humans, but *Candida albicans* is the most common. These yeasts normally live on the skin and mucous membranes in people and are generally harmless. If conditions in the body shift to create an environment favorable to *Candida* overgrowth, infections of the mouth, vagina, urinary tract, skin, or stomach can set in. Most causes of *Candida* overgrowth result from certain drugs, pregnancy, bacterial infections, excess weight, or an overburdened immune system. Vaginal yeast infections, white lesions on the tongue or inner cheek, painful cracks in the skin at the corners of the mouth, or crusted skin rashes around the fingers, toes, or groin are symptoms of candidiasis.

Antifungal drugs are commonly prescribed for up to two weeks. Reducing sugar and yeast products in the diet and taking probiotics are popular complementary approaches to assist in eliminating candidiasis. Daily consumption of curcumin can be added to these alternative methods. The antifungal activity of curcumin was confirmed against fourteen different strains of *Candida*, including *Candida albicans*.[20] It was not as effective as fluconazole—used to prevent and treat fungal infections—but can certainly be used in combination with it to lower the dosage or duration of its use.

9. CARDIOMYOPATHY

Cardiomyopathy is a disease of the heart muscle that causes it to become enlarged, rigid, or thick. The walls and ventricles weaken, making it harder to pump blood. Some people do not experience any symptoms and may not need medical intervention, while others suffer shortness of breath, fatigue, dizziness, irregular heartbeat, chest pain, or swelling in the legs, arms, abdomen, and ankles. There are different types of cardiomyopathies. Hypertrophic cardiomyopathy is the most common and affects one in every five hundred people. This type can be inherited from previous generations or develop over time as a complication of aging, heart conditions, or diseases like diabetes. Other types of cardiomyopathy develop from nutritional deficiencies, drug and alcohol use, certain infections, metabolic disorders, or pregnancy complications. Treatment depends on the type and severity of the disease and includes medication, nonsurgical procedures, surgical implants, or even a heart transplant.

The goal of treatment is to manage symptoms, prevent the condition from getting worse, and lower the risk of complications. Curcumin is a powerful antioxidant that can reduce oxidative stress that damages the heart muscle. Diabetic rats treated with curcumin for one month lessened oxidative damage to the heart and decreased the levels of certain inflammatory enzymes and those involved in blood vessel abnormalities.[21] Another study in diabetic rats found that curcumin prevented an increase in molecular markers indicative of heart enlargement compared to controls not given curcumin.[22] Daily consumption of curcumin can reduce

HEALTH
WELLNESS
BEAUTY
CRAFTS

oxidative stress and perhaps help prevent heart muscle damage in those at risk for this disease.

10. CATARACTS

The most common cause of vision loss in people over the age of forty is from cataracts. These develop when the natural lens of the eye clouds over. This can be a gradual process that happens with aging, or it can be a complication of certain medications or diseases, such as diabetes. In these cases, the lens is often affected more rapidly. Proteins in the lens begin to break down and clump together, causing the cloudiness. Light scatters when it enters the eye rather than focusing on the retina. The symptoms that result include blurred vision, double vision, dulled colors, impaired night vision, and sensitivity to lights. It is like looking through fog or a dirty windshield. If vision is only minimally impaired, new eyeglasses may be all that's needed. If, however, diminished vision is impacting your daily life, cataract surgery may be required. This is a simple, painless procedure that replaces the cloudy lens with an artificial, clear one. Most of those undergoing this surgery regain all or most of their vision.

One theory explaining the development of cataracts is oxidative damage to the lens. Turmeric and curcumin are potent antioxidants and have been proposed as protective agents in preventing or slowing cataract formation. One of the complications of diabetes is the development of cataracts. Diabetic-induced rats were treated with varying concentrations of curcumin or turmeric over an eight-week period. Both substances slowed the progression of cataracts in the treatment groups compared to the rats in the placebo group. The oxidative stress induced by the diabetic state was reversed, and the proteins were prevented from clumping together. Interestingly, turmeric was more effective than curcumin, its most active constituent.[23] Taking turmeric each day may delay the onset of age-related cataract development and be particularly useful for diabetics at risk for this condition.

11. CHOLECYSTITIS

Cholecystitis is an inflammation of the gallbladder, the small organ located beneath the liver. It holds bile produced by the liver and releases it into the small intestine to digest fats. Often, gallstones develop and block the duct leading bile out of the gallbladder. Bile builds up and causes inflammation. A tumor or scar tissue may also cause the same type of obstruction. Symptoms are most apparent after a meal and include severe pain or tenderness in the upper right abdomen, nausea, vomiting, and fever. Reducing inflammation is necessary, so fasting is often recommended to take the stress off the gallbladder. If infection sets in, a course of antibiotics and pain medication are prescribed. Some cases require surgical removal of the gallbladder. After this, the bile will flow from the liver directly to the small intestine. The gallbladder is not an essential organ, and removing it should not affect daily life.

In 1937, the first documented clinical trial using curcumin was published by Oppenheimer. He found that injecting a sodium curcumin solution into healthy patients caused a rapid emptying of bile from their gallbladders. In sixty-seven patients with cholecystitis, oral administration of curcumin over a three-week period cured all but one patient without any ill effects observed.[24] One of the reasons gallstones form is from incomplete or infrequent emptying of the gallbladder. Curcumin prevents this issue and removes the risk of gallstone formation and inflammation.

12. CHRONIC OBSTRuCTIVE PULMONARY DISEASE (CoPD)

This disease is caused by chronic inflammation of the lungs that obstructs airflow and makes breathing difficult. Its two main conditions are emphysema, in which the lung's air sacs are damaged, and bronchitis, characterized by inflamed lining of the bronchial tubes and mucus overproduction. Exposure to lung irritants over prolonged periods contributes to the development of this disease. Smoking is the most common irritant responsible for COPD. Symptoms include shortness of breath, chest tightness, wheezing, and chronic cough. This disease is progressive and gets worse over time. Mild forms of this disease require little intervention other than smoking cessation. In other cases, medications are needed to relax the muscles in the airways and reduce inflammation. Oxygen therapy can be useful to deliver extra oxygen to the lungs. Portable units are available to use when away from home. In severe cases, surgery is recommended to remove parts of the affected lung. Lung transplants are options for some.

Oxidative stress can cause inflammation of the lungs and make breathing more difficult in those with COPD. In addition, this stress on the lungs can lessen the effectiveness of inhaled corticosteroid medications intended to open the airways. Curcumin was shown to restore the activity of an enzyme needed for inhaled corticosteroid medications to work properly.[25] This enzyme is often reduced under oxidative stress, hindering the medications' efficacy. In those with COPD, adding turmeric or curcumin supplements to their daily diet may increase the usefulness of their corticosteroid medications to alleviate their breathing.

13. COLORECTAL POLYPS

Colorectal polyps are small clumps of cells that grow in the inner lining of the colon; they can be tubular, flat, or mushroom shaped. They are very common, and their prevalence increases with age. More than one-third of people over the age of sixty have at least one polyp. They vary in number, size, and location. The most common type is called an adenoma polyp. This type has the potential to develop into cancer. The larger it is, the more likely it is that it will develop into cancer. Having three or more of these polyps, even if benign, increases the probability that future polyps will develop and be cancerous. Some heredity disorders, such as familial adenomatous polyposis (FAP), causes hundreds to thousands of polyps, usually in the teenage years. If not treated, they will very likely develop into cancer. Most polyps do not present with symptoms and are discovered during routine colonoscopies. In some cases, however, blood in the stool, black stools, or iron deficiency anemia may indicate the presence of one or more polyps. They can be removed by endoscopy during bowel examination and analyzed by a pathologist to determine if they are malignant. In FAP, surgery to remove the colon and rectum is sometimes needed. Currently, non-steroidal anti-inflammatories are used because they have been shown to reduce or prevent the formation of polyps. The side effects of these drugs are concerning, however, and include gastro-intestinal bleeding and cardiovascular implications.

With the high incidence of polyp formation and its generally silent presence, taking measures to prevent the formations of polyps seems wise. To reduce the serious side effects caused by non-steroidal anti-inflammatories, try taking curcumin and quercetin, plant polyphenols that are also available as dietary supplements. In five patients with FAP, 480 mg of curcumin and 20 mg of quercetin were given orally three times a day for six months. The number of polyps decreased by an average of 60 percent and the size of the polyps decreased by an average of nearly 51 percent compared to the number and size before treatment.[26] This efficacy combined with the safety of these natural products provides an attractive alternative to current treatments.

14. CROHN'S DISEASE

Crohn's disease is a chronic inflammatory bowel disease affecting sections of the lining of the digestive tract, particularly the deep tissue of the small bowel and beginning of the colon. Symptoms develop gradually and can flare up suddenly and disappear for periods of time. Many people with Crohn's suffer from stomach pain and cramps, diarrhea, poor appetite, rectal bleeding, fatigue, and fever. While some with Crohn's disease find it runs in their family, most discover no such genetic link. The cause is unknown, but viral or bacterial infections may trigger the immune system, setting off an abnormal response causing the immune system to attack cells of the digestive tract. In severe cases, surgery is some-times needed, but most patients are treated with anti-inflammatory or immune-suppressing drugs to reduce inflammation or antibiotics to kill harmful intestinal bacteria.

This disease can be very debilitating and severely impact the quality of life of those afflicted. In some cases, medications don't completely reduce or prevent flare-ups. Curcumin has been shown to work with these medications to improve symptoms. Five patients diagnosed with Crohn's disease were treated over three months with curcumin. In the first month, 360 mg of curcumin was given three times a day. For the second two months, 360 mg of curcumin was given four times a day. Four of the five patients had fewer and less severe symptoms and lower inflammatory activity. They reported more formed stools, fewer trips to the bathroom, and decreased abdominal pain and cramps.[27]

15. DIABETES

Diabetes is a disease that affects the way the body handles glucose, resulting in high levels of this sugar in the blood. There is type 1 diabetes, in which the pancreas produces little or no insulin, type 2 diabetes, in which the pancreas does produce insulin but the body doesn't use it as well as it should, and gestational diabetes, a form of high blood sugar affecting pregnant women. Some people are genetically predisposed to diabetes, but being overweight is also a risk factor. Feelings of thirst, frequent urination, fatigue, tingling, numbness in the hands or feet, and blurry vision are all signs of diabetes. Managing diabetes involves exercising, improving diet, and monitoring blood glucose levels. For many, daily insulin injections are needed.

Hyperglycemia is the hallmark sign of diabetes. Diabetics have to closely monitor their blood sugar levels to ensure they are not too high. Elevated levels can cause damage to the cells lining the blood vessels. Keeping these cells alive and healthy is vitally important because they are necessary to supply blood to the body and are instrumental in tissue growth and repair.

Patients with type 2 diabetes were randomized to receive either 150 mg of curcumin a day for eight weeks, atorvastatin (a statin used to treat blood vessel problems), or a placebo. Those in the curcumin and atorvastatin groups saw significant improvement in the function of the blood vessel cells, but the curcumin group's effect was more beneficial.[28] In healthy subjects, 6 grams of turmeric increased insulin levels after meals,[29] suggesting turmeric may influence the pancreas to secrete more insulin. This effect was later confirmed by another study in prediabetic patients given either curcumin or placebo capsules for nine months. Those receiving curcumin were protected from progressing from the prediabetic state to type 2 diabetes. This may be explained, in part, by the fact that the function of β-cells (which produce, store, and release insulin from the pancreas) was improved in the curcumin treatment group.[30]

Curcumin doesn't just increase insulin secretion and protect important tissue from damage. It has been known for decades to modulate blood sugar levels in diabetic patients.[31] More recently, it was discovered that turmeric fed to diabetic mice was able to significantly suppress an increase in blood glucose levels. This effect was not seen in the diabetic mice fed a non-supplemented diet. Moreover, it was not just curcumin in turmeric but a class of compounds known as sesquiterpenoids that was responsible for this effect.[32]

Some complications of diabetes include cataracts (see page 20), high cholesterol (see page 35), encephalopathy (see next section), kidney disease (see page 39), microangiopathy (see page 45), and retinopathy (see page 54). All these conditions can be helped by curcumin and are discussed within this book.

16. ENCEPHALOPATHY, AS A COMPLICATION OF DIABETES

This is a disease that affects the function or structure of the brain and alters the mental state. It is a potential complication of diabetes that can happen when blood sugar dips too low or rises too high, damaging nerves in the brain. It induces both mental and physical changes in the brain and can cause confusion, memory loss, lethargy, personality changes, poor coordination, tremors, and seizures. Each case is unique, so treatment varies from person to person. If symptoms warrant it, dementia or Alzheimer's prescription drugs can be used.

Maintaining normal blood sugar levels is imperative to prevent nerve damage in the brain. Curcumin fed to diabetic rats significantly abated cognitive decline, oxidative stress, and inflammation in the brain.[33] It may be used in combination with diabetic therapy in the prevention and treatment of diabetic encephalopathy.

17. ENDOTHELIAL DYSFUNCTION

Endothelial cells layer the surface of the inner lining of the blood vessels and are responsible for maintaining blood flow and tissue homeostasis in the vascular system by responding to physical and chemical signals. When their functions are compromised, inflammation and atherosclerosis begin. Diabetes is associated with abnormalities of endothelial function by affecting cell signaling and enzyme activity of endothelial cells. Hyperglycemia, a common state in diabetes, also plays a role in endothelial dysfunction by increasing oxidative stress and decreasing the production of vasodilator molecules, which can increase tension in the arteries.

The influence of dietary factors on vitality and health is often underestimated. Curcumin has many potent actions in the body and resultantly was tested for its efficacy to improve endothelial function. Patients randomly received 300 mg of curcumin, 10 mg of atorvastatin (a drug used to reduce blood vessel problems), or a placebo each day for eight weeks. Both the curcumin and atorvastatin groups improved endothelial function, with the effect being more pronounced in the curcumin group.[34] Atorvastatin's common side effects include diarrhea, joint pain, nasopharyngitis, and hemorrhagic stroke. To avoid these side effects but still improve endothelial function, try taking curcumin instead.

··

18. EPILEPSY

Epilepsy is a disorder of the central nervous system affecting nerve activity in the brain. Groups of nerves can send out the wrong signal and result in a seizure. Some seizures are small and can go unnoticed, while others involve violent muscle contractions and loss of consciousness. Altered emotions and perceptions are common and may cause strange behavior for brief periods. Genetics plays a role in some types of epilepsy, making the person more sensitive to particular triggers that can cause seizures. Brain damage or head injuries may also cause this condition, but in about half of epileptic patients, no known cause has been identified. Doctors generally treat epilepsy with medication to reduce the frequency and intensity of seizures. These medications come with a list of side effects from mild fatigue to severe suicidal thoughts and behaviors. Surgery is warranted in some cases, but this, as always, comes with inherent risks.

Nitric oxide may play a central role in epilepsy by acting as a messenger in the central nervous system and by modulating brain function. Too much nitric oxide in the brain can induce neurotoxicity. Reducing high levels in epileptic rat models was shown to provide an anticonvulsant effect.[35] Complexes of curcumin from turmeric were administered to rats with induced high nitric oxide levels. These complexes were able to reverse nitric oxide levels to normal concentrations, presumably through their antioxidant activities. They significantly lowered nerve cell death and can be used to protect the brain from nitric oxide–induced damage, as observed in epilepsy.[36]

19. ESCHERICHIA COLI

Escherichia coli (E. coli) is a bacterium that normally lives in the intestines of humans and animals. Many types of *E. coli* are harmless and are important to the health of the digestive tract. Several species, however, are pathogenic and cause bloody diarrhea, urinary tract infections, anemia, or kidney failure. Contraction of *E. coli* can be made from contact with infected persons or animals or from consuming food or water containing the bacteria. *E. coli* can contaminate meat during processing, and if it is not cooked to 160 degrees Fahrenheit (71 degrees Celsius), it can survive and infect the consumer. Sometimes cows spread the bacteria to their milk as it passes their udders. If the milk is not pasteurized, the bacteria will continue to live and pose a threat. Even raw fruits and vegetables can have *E. coli* bacteria from contact with contaminated water or people. Three or four days after ingesting *E. coli*, food poisoning becomes evident as symptoms develop. Symptoms usually subside on their own after about a week.

Food poisoning is absolutely miserable. Prevention is best, so cooking meats to their proper temperature and washing produce to remove any offending pathogens are essential. If the bacteria do find their way into a person's intestinal system, consuming turmeric or curcumin can decrease the severity or duration of the illness. Curcumin can increase the destruction of *E. coli* bacteria by elevating levels of a protein involved in mediating the cell death response.[37] It also damages *E. coli* membranes, causing them to leak their contents.[38] This inactivates the bacteria and prevents their replication and spread.

. . . .

20. GENITAL HERPES

More than one in every six people in the United States between the ages of 14 to 49 have genital herpes.[39] This is a viral infection, mainly from the herpes simplex virus type 2 (HSV-2), and less commonly from the herpes simplex virus type 1 (HSV-1). It is spread through sexual contact and is highly contagious. Many people don't know they have the virus because they display little to no symptoms. If symptoms are present, they may include itching and pain in the genital area and sores that look like small red or white bumps that can rupture and ooze, eventually scabbing over. Repeated outbreaks are common, but symptoms are usually milder after the initial outbreak. There is no cure for genital herpes. Treatment with antiviral medications can help heal sores more quickly and lessen the frequency of recurrences. They can also minimize the chance of passing the virus to others. This is particularly important since the virus can be transmitted in the presence or absence of visible sores.

Medications for genital warts are only available through prescription. An alternative that is easily accessible and cost-effective is turmeric. Turmeric contains two antiviral compounds, curcumin and eugenol. These compounds were able to protect mice against genital HSV-2 infection. Eugenol was more effective, and further studies showed significant protection in guinea pigs as well.[40]

TURMERIC OIL FOR VIRAL OUTBREAKS

1. Make a paste of 1 teaspoon of coconut oil mixed with 1/2 tea-spoon of turmeric powder.
2. Apply to the infected area. The coconut oil will melt, so don't put too much on or it will drip.
3. Allow it to sit for 30 minutes. Wash off. Repeat as necessary. The combination of turmeric and coconut oil should halt the viral outbreak and allow healing to begin. Because these compounds are also anti-inflammatory, pain and swelling should also be reduced.

21. GINGIVITIS

Gingiva is the part of the gum around the base of the teeth that becomes diseased and causes gingivitis. The gums tend to bleed easily, become puffy, and turn from pink to red. They begin to recede, and tooth decay sets in. Gingivitis is caused when hardened plaque, called tartar, forms below and above the gum line. Tartar is full of bacteria, and it is the bacteria that begin the infection. Plaque is formed daily on the teeth, but it can easily be removed through daily brushing and flossing. If it is left to harden into tartar, it is much harder to eliminate. This disease is common, and symptoms are often mild, so most people don't know they have it. Professional teeth cleaning is needed, followed by a good oral hygiene routine at home.

Turmeric can be used as an antibacterial agent in mouthwash to prevent the build-up of bacteria in the mouth and the subsequent development of plaque and tartar. A turmeric mouthwash was compared to an antimicrobial commercial mouthwash known to decrease bacteria and reduce swelling, redness, and bleeding. Comparable and significant reductions in bacteria were observed in both mouthwashes.[41] This suggests turmeric can be used alongside daily brushing and flossing for an effective and low-cost approach to managing gingivitis.

TURMERIC MOUTHWASH

1. Boil 5 grams of ground turmeric with two cloves and two dried guava leaves in a cup of water.[42]
2. When the solution has cooled to a comfortable temperature, swish a small amount around the mouth. Pain relief should be immediate.

22. HEPATITIS B

This is an infection caused by the hepatitis B virus. It is most commonly transmitted from mother to baby during birth but can also be acquired through sexual contact or from sharing syringes and needles. Most adults who contract this virus have acute hepatitis B, a short-term illness. Some will feel ill for several weeks with nausea, diarrhea, fatigue, jaundice, and abdominal pain. A small portion of adults and the majority of babies and children with the virus progress to chronic hepatitis B. This long-term illness can lead to cirrhosis and liver cancer. Acute hepatitis B has no treatment other than methods to make the person feel comfortable until the illness passes. Oral antiviral medications can be taken to suppress the virus in chronic cases and slow the progression of liver disease. Prevention can be achieved by taking the hepatitis B vaccine in a three- or four-dose schedule.

Sometimes vaccines are not available, accessible, or desired for hepatitis B prevention. If the virus is contracted, antiviral medication is ideal. Many people, however, are never diagnosed or have limited treatments options depending on their geographic location or financial situation. For these people, obtaining such medications is not feasible. Turmeric is widely available and can be used as a preventative against or for the treatment of hepatitis B. Extracts of turmeric were able to inhibit viral replication in liver cells without having any toxic effects on the liver cells themselves.[43] This suggests adding turmeric to the diet of chronic sufferers or taking curcumin supplements may slow the progression of the infection and protect the liver.

23. HEPATITIS C

Hepatitis C is a viral disease that affects the liver. It is contracted through contaminated blood and can live in the body for many years before symptoms begin to appear. Most people do not know they have hepatitis C until the virus begins to damage the liver and symptoms develop, such as fever, nausea, diarrhea, poor appetite, fatigue, jaundice, muscle aches, and bleeding issues. About 25 percent of cases in the acute phase resolve themselves without treatment. The rest can be treated with antiviral medications to clear the virus from the system. Most cases left untreated, however, will develop into a chronic illness that can cause scarring of the liver, which impairs its function, liver cancer, or even liver failure.

If the liver is too damaged or low-functioning, a liver transplant may be required.

There is no vaccination for hepatitis C as there is for hepatitis A and B. If contracted, most people need antiviral treatment to eliminate the illness or manage their symptoms. While there are many antiviral drugs available for treatment, curcumin from turmeric can be used as a readily available and inexpensive way to clear the infection. It has been shown to inhibit the replication of the hepatitis C virus in laboratory experiments.[44] This demonstrates potential to be used as a natural, non-prescription antiviral agent in humans without the detrimental side effects of prescription antiviral drugs.

24. HIGH CHOLESTEROL

Cholesterol is a waxy, fat-like substance found in cells. It is necessary for the body to make vitamin D, hormones, and bile acids that help digest food. We produce cholesterol on our own, but we also get it in saturated fat and cholesterol-laden foods. It comes in two forms: the good, high-density lipoprotein cholesterol (HDL), and the bad, LDL. High cholesterol is when there are high levels of cholesterol in the blood, both HDL and LDL. When there is too much LDL cholesterol in the body, however, it can build up in the arteries and increase the chances of getting coronary heart disease. Plaque containing cholesterol builds up inside the arteries and cause partial or full blockage, leading to narrowing and hardening of the arteries. This can lead to a heart attack or stroke. Statins are drugs commonly prescribed to lower LDL cholesterol. Taking statins can cause intestinal problems and muscle inflammation.

Cholesterol levels respond well to changes in diet. Eating foods low in saturated fats and reducing intake of animal products, which are the contributors of cholesterol in the diet, will do wonders. Adding turmeric to the diet can counter high cholesterol levels and perhaps be used in place of statins to improve lipid profiles. An extract of turmeric was given twice a day to one group of overweight participants with high blood fat levels. A second group with similar clinical parameters was given placebo. After three months, the turmeric-treated group had significantly reduced their LDL cholesterol as well as their very low-density lipoprotein cholesterol (VLDL) and triglyceride levels. This effect was not seen in the placebo group.[45] Curcumin isolated from turmeric exhibited similar results to the turmeric extract. Patients with acute coronary syndrome, of which high blood cholesterol is a risk factor, were given three different doses of curcumin over a one-year period. LDL cholesterol levels significantly decreased, and HDL cholesterol levels significantly increased. Interestingly, the lower the dose, the higher the effect.[46] It appears 15 milligrams of curcumin administered three times a day is sufficient to reduce LDL cholesterol levels and improve the cardiovascular condition.

25. HUMAN PAPILLOMAVIRUS (HPV)

More than 100 varieties of human papillomavirus (HPV) exist, and over 79 million Americans currently have some form of this virus.[47] These viruses cause plantar warts, common warts, genital warts, and flat warts. Thirteen types of HPV, however, can cause cancer. Of these, cervical cancer is the most common, but cancers of the anus, penis, vagina, and throat have also been associated with certain strains of HPV. These high-risk types are transmitted through sexual contact, and most sexually active men and women have been infected with HPV at some point during their lives. Most infections clear up on their own. Only a small portion of these infections, with high-risk types of the virus, progress to cancer. HPV types 16 and 18 are responsible for 70 percent of precancerous cervical lesions and cervical cancer. This slow-growing cancer can take fifteen to twenty years to develop. Symptoms only appear after the disease has advanced and can include abnormal vaginal bleeding, pelvic pain, vaginal discharge, one swollen leg, and fatigue. Vaccines have recently been developed to prevent high-risk HPV infections. They are targeted towards girls who have not yet become sexually active and, more recently, to boys to protect against genital cancers and genital warts.

Regular pap smears or HPV tests can help determine infection. If positive, curcumin may be used as a therapeutic intervention that is both effective and safe at clearing the virus. A vaginal polycream containing curcumin as one of the ingredients and a curcumin vaginal capsule were given to HPV-positive women. Placebo creams and capsules were administered to two control groups. After thirty days, the polycream cleared the virus in almost 88 percent of women while the curcumin capsules cleared the virus in a higher number of cases than the placebo group, although not significantly.[48] Curcumin also proved to be cytotoxic to HPV-associated cervical cancer cells through nuclear fragmentation and inhibition of expression of two viral oncogenes. The response was both time- and dose-dependent.[49] It looks like curcumin can be

HEALTH

WELLNESS

BEAUTY

CRAFTS

beneficial at various stages of HPV infection, from early clearance to later tumor management.

26. HUNTINGTON'S DISEASE

Huntington's disease (HD) is a genetic disorder caused by a defect in a single gene. It only takes one copy of this gene to be present for the disease to develop. In addition, each person has a 50 percent chance of passing this gene, and the disease, on to their offspring. Currently, about 30,000 Americans have Huntington's. Symptoms of mental and physical deterioration usually begin between the ages of thirty and fifty and get progressively worse over the next ten to twenty-five years. The course of the disease is different for everyone, but some of the common symptoms are involuntary muscle movements, impaired balance and gait, slurred speech, difficulty swallowing, impaired judgement, forgetfulness, depression, and personality changes. In some cases, children and teens develop the disease. There is no cure or treatment to alter the course, but working with speech language pathologists and physical and occupational therapists can help manage some of the physical symptoms. Medications to control movements and help with mood disorders are also commonly prescribed.

Treatments for neurodegeneration resulting from HD need to be developed that avoid the side effects of current therapies. Curcumin has the ability to cross the blood-brain barrier where it can exercise neuroprotective activity. In a fruit fly model of HD, dietary curcumin reduced symptoms of the disease by suppressing cell death and neuronal degeneration, events that lead to the progression of Huntington's.[50] In a rat model of Huntington's, curcumin encapsulated in solid lipid nanoparticles improved muscular movements and coordination.[51] When curcumin was combined with black pepper to enhance bioavailability, motor movements in another rat HD model were enhanced, and biochemical and neurochemical irregularities were improved.[52] Curcumin looks to be a promising therapeutic intervention that can slow the progression of symptoms without any detrimental side effects.

27. KIDNEY DISEASE, AS A COMPLICATION OF DIABETES

This type of kidney disease develops in up to 40 percent of patients with type 1 and type 2 diabetes. Kidneys filter out waste products and extra fluid from the body. When the blood has high levels of glucose, the kidneys wind up filtering too much blood. Over time, they become overworked, and the blood vessels, along with their filtering ability, become damaged. This causes a build-up of fluids and wastes in the body. In the beginning stages, symptoms may not be noticeable because the kidneys are working very hard to make up for any loss of function. As the disease progresses and kidney activity is greatly diminished, signs begin to develop. Fluid build-up and swelling of the hands and feet are often the first indicators of kidney disease. These are commonly followed by nausea, vomiting, confusion, an increased need to urinate, protein in the urine, and fatigue. To prevent kidney disease or slow its progression, diabetics should keep blood glucose levels in their target range and maintain a healthy blood pressure. Sometimes medications can be prescribed to control high blood pressure or high blood sugar, lower cholesterol, or control protein in the urine.

Turmeric can provide protection to the kidneys so that they continue to filter out wastes and keep fluid levels in the body at normal levels. Patients with type 2 diabetes were either given 500 mg of turmeric three times a day or three placebo capsules a day over a two-month period. Compared to pre-study levels, it was found that patients consuming turmeric had significantly lower levels of protein in their urine and lower levels of inflammation-inducing compounds. Turmeric was found to be safe in all patients, with no side effects being reported.[53]

28. LISTERIOSIS

Listeriosis is a serious infection caused by eating food contaminated with the bacteria *Listeria monocytogenes*. These bacteria are contracted by humans most commonly through deli meats, hot dogs, unpasteurized milk, and soft cheeses. Most people who come into contact with these bacteria are not seriously affected and may experience muscle aches, headaches, nausea, and diarrhea. Pregnant mothers need to be very vigilant during pregnancy because *Listeria* can be life-threatening to the fetus and newborn baby. People with weakened immune systems are also at higher risk of developing serious or life-threatening complications. This illness usually runs its course without intervention, but in high-risk patients, antibiotics are commonly prescribed.

Listeria bacteria contain a pore-forming protein that allows the bacteria to escape into the cytoplasm of cells, where it grows rapidly and cannot be detected by the host's immune system. Infected cells treated with curcumin targeted this protein and decreased the bacteria's escape into the cytoplasm of the host cell, thereby limiting its growth. In animal studies, curcumin increased protection against *Listeria* infection and helped the animals clear the bacteria out of their system.[54] Consuming turmeric or curcumin supplements may help speed recovery and lessen the severity of symptoms.

29. LUNG CANCER

The lungs bring oxygen into the body with each breath of air and release carbon dioxide with each exhale. People who smoke, breathe in secondhand smoke, are chronically exposed to environmental irritants, or have a family history of lung cancer should be concerned about this disease. Smoking is the number one cause of lung cancer and is the leading cause of cancer death in the United States.

Lung cancer can occur when the cells lining the lungs become damaged. Over time, they no longer function normally, and cancer can develop. There are two major types of lung cancers: small cell, a rapidly spreading cancer comprising up to 15 percent of lung cancers, and non-small cell, the most common type, afflicting about 85 percent of those with a positive diagnosis. There are few symptoms in the early stages, but as it progresses, lung cancer can cause chronic cough, wheezing, chest pain, headache, and the coughing up of blood. Treatment depends on the stage of cancer and the overall health of the individual. Chemotherapy, radiation, and surgery are common options to eradicate this disease.

Curcumin is known to have anticarcinogenic properties. Curcumin, together with another turmeric compound, quercetin, were investigated for their ability to protect mice against the effects of lung cancer. These phytochemicals were given in drinking water to lung cancer–induced mice. Lipid peroxidation activity and reactive oxygen species levels were reduced while important antioxidant levels were increased.[55] These changes protect cells from damage and interfere with the cancer's progression. Curcumin is an inexpensive and effective way prevent or slow the advancement of lung cancer in the at-risk population.

30. LUPUS NEPHRITIS

Systemic lupus erythematosus is an autoimmune disease that affects the kidneys, skin, joints, and brain. The body's immune system attacks its own healthy tissues, and in the case of lupus nephritis, it attacks the kidneys. Most people diagnosed with lupus are women. The cause is not definitively known, but family history, infections, and chemical pollutants are suspected. Lupus nephritis is characterized by inflammation of the blood vessels that filter out wastes and extra fluid from the body. Signs and symptoms vary, but some include protein and blood in the urine, weight gain, and fluid build-up in the body. Drugs that suppress the body's immune response to prevent it from attacking the kidneys are often prescribed. Other drugs are used to reduce blood pressure in an attempt to lower protein loss or remove excess fluid to decrease tissue swelling.

Treatments of lupus nephritis can be expensive, and they do not always work. Turmeric can provide a safe and inexpensive way to combat the symptoms of this disease and may be especially useful as an alternative when other treatments have failed. Patients with lupus nephritis were given 1,500 mg of turmeric a day for three months. A control group receiving the same number of placebo capsules was established. After three months, the patients consuming turmeric had significant decreases in the amount of blood and protein in their urine. No such effect was noted in the placebo group.[56] This suggests turmeric improves the functioning of the kidneys and can be used as a safe and effective natural alternative to expensive medications.

31. MALARiA

The bite of a female *Anopheles* mosquito infected with Plasmodium parasites transmits these parasites to humans. The parasites enter the bloodstream and travel to the liver, where they begin to multiply. Some malarial parasites remain in the liver, and others are released into the bloodstream. They infect red blood cells and continue to grow and multiply inside them. Eventually the red blood cells are destroyed and new daughter parasites are released. They continue the cycle by invading other red blood cells. The incubation period lasts an average of ten days, after which time the human host will begin to develop symptoms. Fever, headache, chills, sweats, fatigue, and sometimes seizures begin and can be misdiagnosed as flu, particularly in areas where malaria is uncommon. In the United States, about 1,700 cases are diagnosed each year, most often from travelers returning from countries where malaria is common. Those traveling to malaria-endemic countries should take precautions and get tested immediately if symptoms develop. If left untreated, vital organs can become damaged and, in severe cases, can be fatal. The World Health Organization recommends treatment with artemisinin (sweet wormwood)-based combination therapy (ACT). Sweet wormwood reduces the concentration of the parasite in the bloodstream within the first three days of infection, and other drugs are used to eliminate the rest. Malaria is becoming resistant to ACT treatment, however, with no alternatives to sweet wormwood available. There is a vaccine licensed for use in Europe, but it is not yet available in the United States.

Finding an alternative source to current treatments is becoming more important with the rise in drug resistant strains of the Plasmodium parasite. Two herbs used in Ayurveda and traditional Chinese medicine to protect the liver and reduce fever were tested in combination with curcumin on their anti-malarial activity on drug-resistant and sensitive strains of the malaria-carrying Plasmodium parasite. Curcumin had a synergistic effect with each of these drugs and enhanced the anti-malarial activity in both strains, affecting the replication of the parasite in the red blood cells during the ring stage of development. No toxicity was observed.[57] A new alternative treatment using this herbal combination has shown to be effective in the treatment of malaria.

32. MICROANGIOPATHY, AS A COMPLICATION OF DIABETES

Microangiopathy is a disease of the small blood vessels of the body, and one of the major causes is diabetes. If blood glucose levels are high, the insulin-independent endothelial cells lining the surface of the blood vessels take up more glucose than normal. What eventually results are blood vessel walls that are abnormally thicker and weaker. They begin to leak blood and protein. Blood flow slows, and organs become deprived of oxygen and nutrients. Functional and structural damage follows. The consequences are far reaching and include atherosclerosis, kidney disease, retinopathy, and neuropathy.

Controlling blood sugar levels is the first step in preventing damage to the small blood vessels. Sometimes, despite best efforts, those measures are not enough, and additional therapies need to be considered. Curcumin is known to have anti-inflammatory and other beneficial effects on the endothelial lining of the small blood vessels. Twenty-five patients suffering from diabetic microangiopathy were given a 1-gram formulation of curcumin with enhanced bioavailability each day for four weeks. A comparable control group did not receive curcumin but continued to manage their disease as before. At the end of four weeks, microangiopathy was improved in all subjects receiving the curcumin formulation. A significant decrease in skin blood flux and swelling was noted, allowing an increase in the amount of oxygen dissolved in the blood. No effect on microcirculation was observed in the control group.[58]

33. MIDDLE EAR INFECTION

There are two types of middle ear infection, also called otitis media. Acute otitis media comes on quickly and is accompanied by swelling and redness in the ear. Pain, difficulty hearing, fever, headache, and difficulty sleeping are other symptoms. It is caused when viruses or bacteria enter the middle ear, often through the Eustachian tubes that connect the middle ear to the throat. Respiratory illnesses or allergies can block these tubes, and fluids can accumulate in the middle ear and allow bacteria or viruses to flourish. The second type of middle ear infection is called otitis media with effusion. This is when fluid in the ear persists even after the initial infection has gone away. The ear can feel full or heavy, and hearing is impacted. Most middle ear infections occur in children, affecting 80 percent of them by the time they are three years old. These infections often resolve on their own. In persistent or severe cases, antibiotics are prescribed. To help alleviate pain, a warm compress over the affected ear and over-the-counter pain relievers are helpful.

A major cause of pain and discomfort with middle ear infections stems from inflamed tissue in this space behind the eardrum. Curcumin, a known anti-inflammatory, was tested in rats with acute middle ear infections. It decreased inflammation of tissue in the middle ear and was found to be safe, making it a potential treatment to reduce swelling and pain associated with this infection.[59]

34. MULTIPLE SCLEROSIS

Multiple sclerosis is the body's immune system responding abnormally toward the protective sheath surrounding nerve fibers of the central nervous system as well as to the nerve fibers themselves. Parts of the nerves are damaged, and messages traveling between the brain and spinal cord are interrupted. The cause of multiple sclerosis is still unknown, but environmental factors are thought to trigger the onset in genetically predisposed individuals. Most people are diagnosed between the ages of twenty and fifty, and it is much more common in women than men. The most common disease course is known as relapsing-remitting multiple sclerosis. Relapses with new symptoms are followed by periods of remission in which some or all of the symptoms disappear. Many of these cases progress to secondary progressive multiple sclerosis, in which a steady increase in symptoms are observed over time. Periods of remission are still common. Others experience a progression of symptoms without periods of remission. This is primary progressive multiple sclerosis. Symptoms can vary from one person to another, but common ones include numbness, vision loss, double vision, lack of coordination, tremors, and slurred speech. There is no cure for multiple sclerosis, and treatments are designed to slow the progression of the disease and manage symptoms. Corticosteroids are the preferred drug to reduce nerve inflammation. Side effects are increased blood pressure, mood swings, and insomnia.

Curcumin's anti-inflammatory activity was investigated for its ability to improve symptoms associated with multiple sclerosis. Mice treated with curcumin inhibited a critical molecule that plays a role in damaging the protective sheath surrounding nerve cells.[60] The sheath and underlying fiber remain undamaged and can continue to function normally. This protective action shows promise in slowing the progression of this disease and keeping the patient in remission.

35. OSTEOARTHRITIS

Arthritis is the most common disability in the United States, affecting more than fifty million people. Osteoarthritis is one of the two most common types and is characterized by inflammation of the joints. The joints provide the connection between bones that allow for movement. They are cushioned by cartilage to allow the joint to move smoothly and easily. In osteoarthritis, the cartilage breaks down and causes the inflammation. Extra fluid is produced in the joint, resulting in swelling. This disease affects many people as they age due to natural wear and tear. Heredity plays a role, as does injury from trauma or disease. Those afflicted suffer from joints that are painful, creaky, stiff, and swollen. Their range of motion is reduced, particularly in the hands, feet, spine, hips, and knees. Reducing the stress on the joint cartilage is recommended to alleviate some of the symptoms. This involves losing weight and avoiding certain activities. The goal of treatment is to reduce pain and inflammation to allow for more comfortable movement.

Medications are taken as pills, creams, gels, and even injections into the arthritic joint. Side effects of these can include gastrointestinal distress such as stomach upset, diarrhea, or ulcers.

Potential treatments for osteoarthritis include compounds with anti-inflammatory properties. Curcumin is one such compound that has been found to reduce pain and improve physical function and quality of life.[61] Two hundred milligrams of a curcumin complex was administered each day for three months to fifty patients with osteoarthritis. A decrease in pain and stiffness and an increase in the physical functioning of the joints was noted. Levels of C-reactive protein were decreased, indicating an attenuated anti-inflammatory response.[62] A longer-term study using this same curcumin complex in one hundred patients with osteoarthritis found that curcumin was well tolerated and can be used for long-term treatment.[63]

Curcumin may also able to increase the effectiveness of osteoarthritis drugs. A synergistic effect between curcumin and a popular non-steroidal anti-inflammatory drug was discovered that inhibited the growth of cells that degrade cartilage in the joints.[64] Lower concentrations of these anti-inflammatory drugs may be taken with curcumin to offset the potential cardiovascular toxicity and other side effects that may result from long-term use. Curcumin may also be taken in place of medications that relieve pain. Primary knee osteoarthritis patients were randomized to receive either 1,500 milligrams of turmeric a day or 1,200 milligrams of ibuprofen a day for four weeks. Turmeric was found to be as effective as ibuprofen in treating the symptoms of osteoarthritis but had significantly fewer gastrointestinal upsets.[65]

HEALTH

WELLNESS

BEAUTY

CRAFTS

HEALTH

WELLNESS

BEAUTY

CRAFTS

36. PARKINSON'S

This is a progressive disorder of the central nervous system that can cause tremors, stiffness, slow movement, and loss of balance. Nerve cells become damaged in the brain, causing dopamine levels to drop. This leads to abnormal brain activity that manifests itself in those characteristic symptoms. The cause of Parkinson's disease is largely unknown, but it is believed that genetic predisposition combined with environmental triggers plays a role. As this disease progresses, cognitive function declines, and those afflicted can experience insomnia, depression, constipation, fatigue, or bladder problems. Parkinson's can't be cured, but medications can be taken to improve the symptoms. The medications increase or substitute for dopamine in the brain. Some advanced cases may opt for surgery to implant electrodes in a specific part of the brain to help reduce the symptoms. Exercise, physical therapy, and speech language therapy are often recommended.

Free radicals have been implicated in the development of Parkinson's disease. These are uncharged molecules that are highly reactive and set off a chain reaction in a cell that can destroy it. Antioxidants neutralize free radicals and protect the cell from damage. Curcumin is an antioxidant, and it was shown to exhibit neuroprotective effects in a rat model of Parkinson's disease. Specifically, dopamine levels, which slowly decrease with the progression of Parkinson's, were increased in the part of the brain responsible for automatic movements and cognition.[66] This increase may offset the development or progression of symptoms associated with Parkinson's.

37. PEPTIC uLCERS

Ulcers are holes in the protective lining of the stomach, small intestine, and esophagus. Sores develop that may cause stomach pain, bloating, heartburn, nausea, and fatty food intolerance. Infection with *H. pylori* is thought to be the main cause. Overuse of painkillers, smoking, stress, and heavy alcohol use are other contributing factors. If *H. pylori* are present, treatment involves a course of antibiotics to kill the bacteria. Medications to neutralize, block, or reduce the production of stomach acid are often prescribed. It is imperative that the use of painkillers, smoking, and alcohol is greatly reduced or stopped.

Turmeric is able to heal peptic ulcers. Seventy-six percent of patients with duodenal or gastric ulcers saw complete resolution of their condition after twelve weeks of turmeric treatment. This result was achieved through five daily doses of 600 milligrams of turmeric capsules. No significant changes were seen in blood chemistry or liver or kidney function.[67] Even much smaller doses, such as 1 gram of turmeric per day, can reduce gastric ulcers in a comparable manner.[68] Turmeric appears to be safe and effective at healing peptic ulcers and their associated symptoms.

38. PERIoDONTITIS

It is extremely important to take have a good oral hygiene routine to prevent periodontitis. This is a serious gum disease in which the gums pull away from the teeth and form pockets where bacteria can breed and cause inflammation. The pockets become deeper, allowing more bacteria to accumulate. Inflammation worsens, and infection sets in. Eventually the gums, tissue, and bones that support the teeth are destroyed, and the teeth may fall out or need to be removed. Be on the lookout for gums that are red, swollen, and tender to the touch. New spaces may develop between the teeth, and the teeth could begin to feel loose. If this happens or if the gums recede or pus is found between the teeth and gums, it is time to take action and see a dentist to stop the progression of this disease.

The growth of different types of bacteria commonly responsible for the development of periodontitis were inhibited by curcumin in a dose-dependent manner. Only very low levels of curcumin were needed to suppress biofilm growth on teeth. *Porphyromonas gingivalis*, the bacteria most responsible for the development of chronic periodontitis, was inhibited by more than 80 percent.[69] Brushing your teeth with turmeric—it surprisingly doesn't stain teeth—or using it in a mouthwash can be part of a daily oral care routine to reduce the growth of bacteria and prevent gum disease. (See Turmeric Mouthwash, page 33.)

39. PROSTATE CANCER

This is cancer that occurs in a man's prostate, the small gland that produces seminal fluid to nourish and transport sperm. It can begin when some cells in the prostate mutate and begin to grow and divide rapidly. They live long after normal prostate cells die and come together to form tumors. These tumors can grow to invade nearby tissue, or some abnormal cells can break off and spread to other parts of the body. Some prostate cancers grow slowly and remain confined to the prostate. These often require minimal treatment and monitoring. Other types can be more aggressive and spread quickly. These need more invasive treatments and usually consist of surgery, chemotherapy, radiation, or hormone therapy. Advanced cases may cause difficulty urinating, slow urine stream, blood in the semen, erectile dysfunction, and bone or pelvic pain.

Curcumin is a powerful agent against tumor formation. Cells treated with curcumin inhibited the expression of a gene that is able to transform healthy cells into cancer cells under certain circumstances. This significantly decreased the formation of prostate cancer cells as well as their movement from one part of the body to another.[70] In human trials, three daily doses of a whole foods formulation containing 100 milligrams of turmeric powder—along with broccoli powder, pomegranate whole fruit powder, and green tea extract—was able to significantly prevent an increase in prostate-specific antigen levels.[71] These are proteins produced in the prostate gland that often show elevated levels in the blood of men with prostate cancer. Although each ingredient in the whole foods formulation may have played a role in preventing or slowing the progression of prostate cancer, turmeric's demonstrated anticancer reputation makes it likely a key contributor to the magnitude of this outcome.

40. RETINOPATHY, AS A COMPLICATION OF DIABETES

One of the many complications of diabetes is damage to the light-sensitive retina at the back of the eye. Over time, too much sugar in the blood can damage the blood vessels in the retina, causing them to leak blood and other fluids. The retinal tissue swells, and vision becomes cloudy and blurry. Some people notice spots or dark strings floating across their vision or have difficulty seeing at night. Retinopathy is progressive and commonly affects both eyes. Early stages of this disease often have no symptoms and require little treatment other than controlling blood glucose levels. As more blood vessels become blocked and nourishment to the retina decreases, the disease advances to proliferative diabetic retinopathy. Because of the extent of damage to the blood vessels, new blood vessels in the retina begin to grow. These are abnormal, however, and leak into the gel-like substance that fills the eye. Vision can become partially or fully blocked. Laser treatments to stop the leakage of blood and fluid or shrink abnormal blood vessels can help restore some vision. Surgery to remove blood and scar tissue from the eye is also available.

Oxidative stress and inflammation are also thought to contribute to the development of diabetic retinopathy. Because of its antioxidant and anti-inflammatory properties, curcumin was investigated as a compound to prevent the progression of these processes in the retinas of rats. Diabetic rats were supplemented with either cur-cumin or placebo over a six-week period. In the curcumin group, antioxidant activity was preserved, while in the placebo group, antioxidant activity decreased. Curcumin not only decreased oxidative stress, but markers for inflammation and cell damage were reduced.[72] Curcumin has a beneficial effect on maintaining favorable conditions in the eye to prevent or slow the progression of diabetic retinopathy.

41. RHEUMATOID ARTHRITIS

Rheumatoid arthritis is an autoimmune disorder in which the immune system mistakenly attacks its own body tissues. The lining of the joints become painfully swollen and can lead to bone erosion and joint deformity over time. Symptoms can spread to other non-joint tissues of the body. It's not known what causes this disease, but genetics combined with environmental triggers are suspected. This chronic disease is without a cure and is managed mostly through medications. Non-steroidal anti-inflammatory drugs, steroids, or disease-modifying antirheumatic drugs can be prescribed to reduce pain, swelling, and joint damage. Possible side effects include digestive problems, liver and kidney damage, heart problems, thinning of bones, diabetes, weight gain, and severe lung infections.

The anti-inflammatory activity of turmeric has been known and used for inflammatory disorders for centuries. To this end, the effectiveness of curcumin was demonstrated in a small number of patients almost forty years ago.[73] A more recent study showed that

500 milligrams of curcumin was more effective in reducing the signs and symptoms of rheumatoid arthritis than 50 milligrams of diclofenac sodium, a common non-steroidal anti-inflammatory drug used to treat inflammation and pain.[74] Animal studies indicate that in order for curcumin to work, it must be taken before the onset of inflammation.[75]

42. RIFT VALLEY FEVER

Rift Valley fever is a viral disease primarily observed in domesticated livestock, but it can be transmitted to humans through direct or indirect contact with the blood or organs of infected animals. Farmers, veterinarians, slaughterhouse workers, and herders are at higher risk of infection. The virus must enter the human host through broken skin, be inhaled into the lungs, or be transmitted by mosquitos. Outbreaks have been reported mainly in sub-Saharan Africa, but Saudi Arabia and Yemen have been more recent targets, indicating that the virus is spreading. In those exposed to the virus, symptoms are usually mild and flu-like, with accompanying liver damage, sensitivity to light, and possible joint, neck, and back pain. They last up to a week, with the immune system overcoming the infection. A small percentage develop more severe symptoms, including eye disease, inflammation of the brain, or hemorrhagic fever, which can be fatal. A vaccine has been developed for Rift Valley fever but is not yet licensed and commercially available. Treatment with the antiviral Ribavirin is sometimes used, but its effectiveness is suboptimal. Severe cases are currently managed by supportive care.

Periodically, outbreaks of Rift Valley fever occur that can quickly affect hundreds of people. Natives and visitors to high-risk areas must be aware of this disease, since its diagnosis can be difficult due to its non-specific symptoms, especially early in the development of the infection. Taking curcumin as a preventative—or, if diagnosed with the virus, as a treatment—can help eliminate the virus from the body. Cell cultures infected with the Rift Valley fever virus and treated with curcumin saw significant reductions in levels of the infectious virus. Curcumin directly binds to and inactivates a protein in infected cells that is needed for viral replication. Pretreatment of mice with curcumin for twenty-four hours prior to infection, followed by an additional three days of further curcumin administration, resulted in decreased levels of viral replication in the liver of these animals.[76]

43. SCHIZOPHRENIA

Schizophrenia is a serious mental illness that affects how a person thinks, acts, and feels. It does not mean those afflicted have multiple personalities or violent tendencies. What it is does mean is that schizophrenics may experience hallucinations, delusions, and cognitive issues or become socially withdrawn, apathetic, or emotionally disconnected. One percent of Americans have this disorder. It is usually diagnosed between the late teens to early thirties and can be caused by genetic factors, viral infections, immune disorders, chemical imbalances in the brain, or the formation of abnormal structural pathways during fetal development. Because symptoms are nonspecific, diagnosis can be difficult. Once made,

HEALTH

WELLNESS

BEAUTY

CRAFTS

however, treatment can begin. Recovery and rehabilitation programs help reintegrate people with this illness back into their communities and help them lead independent and well-adjusted lives. Antipsychotic medications can be used to help control the symptoms by reducing biochemical imbalances in the brain. They are known to produce side effects, however, including dry mouth, constipation, dizziness, tremors, and involuntary muscular movements.

Tardive dyskinesia is a side effect of some of the antipsychotic medications prescribed to treat schizophrenia. Chronic use of these medications can cause uncontrollable stiff, jerky movements of the face and body. One of the factors inducing this reaction is oxidative stress. Curcumin, a powerful antioxidant, inhibited drug-induced tongue protrusions, chewing in the absence of food, and facial jerking in rats chronically fed an antipsychotic medication. The response to curcumin was dose-dependent. Curcumin lowered oxidative damage in the rat brains and reversed the decline in dopamine, serotonin, and norepinephrine, neurotransmitters that can change the way an animal—or person—reacts to stimuli.[77]

44. SCLERODERMA

Scleroderma is a chronic disease of the connective tissues that affects about 300,000 Americans. It is more common in women than men and is usually diagnosed between the ages of twenty-five and fifty-five, although children can develop it too. Scleroderma results from an overproduction of collagen, a fibrous protein that gives tissue strength and elasticity. The body's immune system plays a role in this abnormal collagen production, and research has shown there is a susceptibility gene that raises the probability of getting the disease, but it does not cause it. There are two types: localized scleroderma and systemic scleroderma. The first is relatively mild and affects a few places on the skin or muscles, causing waxy patches of thickened skin. It rarely spreads. The second is more comprehensive and affects connective tissue in many parts of the body, including important internal organs. These organs can become hard and fibrous, causing them to lose function. Problems with the skin have been known to improve over time, but damage to the internal organs tends to worsen. There is no cure for scleroderma, but medications may be taken to dilate blood vessels, prevent the symptoms of acid reflux, relieve pain, or suppress the immune system. Physical therapy can help improve strength and mobility.

A disease with no cure must be continuously managed to ensure the best quality of life possible. Taking medications has its toll on the body, and many new symptoms can develop. Using natural products, like turmeric, can help ease symptoms of the disease and cut down on long-term drug use. Curcumin from turmeric may have beneficial value in treating scleroderma. It was shown to induce cell death in scleroderma lung fibroblasts. These are cells that produce abnormally high amounts of collagen. Interestingly, healthy lung fibroblasts were not affected. They maintained their ability to produce normal amounts of collagen.[78] It is hoped that this result will be replicated in fibroblasts from other organs as well.

HEALTH

WELLNESS

BEAUTY

CRAFTS

45. SKIN CANCER

This common form of cancer is the abnormal growth of skin cells resulting from a mutation that allows the cells to grow out of control and form a cancerous mass. It develops most often on the sun-exposed areas of the skin, but it can develop in areas protected from the harmful ultraviolet (UV) radiation of the sun that often causes it. Other factors, such as exposure to toxic chemicals or a weakened immune system, may also be responsible.

There are three types. Basal cell carcinoma appears most often on the face and neck and can look like a waxy bump or scar-like lesion. Squamous cell carcinoma is most frequent in areas of the skin exposed to the sun and can look like a red nodule or a flat lesion with a scaly, crusted surface. Melanomas can appear anywhere and are characterized by large brownish spots with darker speckles or dark lesions on the hands, feet, or mucous membranes. Moles that change in color or size, or that bleed or that have irregular borders, may be melanoma. Surgery, radiation, or topical medications are the conventional treatments for skin cancer.

Curcumin has anticancer properties and can be used as part of a treatment protocol to destroy skin cancer. It has the ability to regulate biological pathways that inhibit melanoma cell migration and invasion to other areas of the body so that the cancer remains localized. It also increases death in melanoma cells.[79] Curcumin was packaged with a gene that encodes a protein playing a key role in cell growth and death and delivered by iontophoresis (movement of particles through the skin using an electric field) to mice with melanoma. Tumor progression was significantly inhibited.

This method was found to be as effective as administering these compounds directly into the tumor.[80]

46. *STAPHYLOCOCCUS* INFECTION

There are over thirty types of bacterial *Staphylococcus* (staph) infections, but most are caused by *Staphylococcus aureus (S. aureus)*. These bacteria are responsible for skin infections, pneumonia, food poisoning, blood poisoning, and toxic shock syndrome. Staph skin infections are most common and are usually minor. They look like pimples, blisters, or boils. More severe infections, however, can show red, swollen rashes with pus or drainage. Many people carry these bacteria on their skin or in their noses without any symptoms. The bacteria get into the skin through cuts or scrapes, so it is important to keep wounds clean and to wash hands regularly. If the bacteria invade the body and get into the bloodstream, infections can turn up in numerous organs and become life threatening. Treatment for minor staph infections is usually a course of antibiotics or drainage of infected areas. Severe infections require hospitalization. Many varieties of staph have become resistant to antibiotics. New treatments are needed to continue to fight these ubiquitous bacteria.

Curcumin has antibiotic properties that extend to *S. aureus*. Most of these strains secrete a cytotoxic protein that can form pores in cellular membranes and is essential for the development and progression of this infection. Curcumin can inhibit membrane rupture from this protein by directly binding to it and rendering it inactive. It was also able to reduce lung cell damage induced by this same protein.[81] Another study exposing *S. aureus* to curcumin demonstrated its antibacterial activity by damaging their cell membranes, leading to leakage.[82]

47. STREP THROAT

Strep throat is a common bacterial infection of the throat and tonsils. The symptoms come on very suddenly and cause a sore, red, inflamed throat with white patches or tiny red spots on the back of the roof of the mouth. It is often accompanied by a fever, tender lymph nodes, and headache. *Streptococcus pyogenes*, or group A streptococcus, is the bacteria responsible for this contagious infection. It is spread when a healthy person inhales contaminated air droplets from the cough or sneeze of an infected person. It can also be acquired from sharing food or drinks. Even touching surfaces can pick up the bacteria and cause illness if the bacteria are transferred to the mouth, nose, or eyes. Once transmitted, it takes two to five days for symptoms to develop. As long as symptoms are present, the infection is contagious. Oral antibiotics are prescribed to shorten the duration of the illness, reduce the risk of spreading the infection to other parts of the body, and prevent the spread of the bacteria to others.

Curcumin is an effective antibacterial against *Streptococcus pyogenes* and can be used to help overcome this infection. It was also found to work synergistically with commonly used antibiotics like ciprofloxacin, gentamicin, vancomycin, and amikacin.[83] The symptoms of strep throat can be resolved sooner, and smaller doses of antibiotics may prove just as effective as the higher amounts.

Turmeric is also an anti-inflammatory and can help reduce swelling and pain while working toward eradicating the bacteria. Add a teaspoon of turmeric to a cup of salt water and gargle every few hours.

48. ULCERATIVE PROCTITIS AND COLITIS

Ulcerative proctitis is a mild form of ulcerative colitis, an inflammatory bowel disease that causes long-lasting inflammation in the innermost lining of the large intestine. In this form of colitis, inflammation is usually limited to the rectum, perhaps spreading a little bit into the colon. The symptoms can vary depending on where the inflammation is located in the large colon and are usually mild to moderate with periods of remission. Some signs are diarrhea with blood or pus, rectal bleeding, abdominal or rectal pain, an urgency or inability to defecate, fever, fatigue, and weight loss. Treatment options include dietary adjustments, immunosuppressants, anti-diarrhea medication, or anti-inflammatory drugs. Severe cases may need surgery to remove the colon and rectum.

Diseases of the colon can make it difficult to travel or even leave the home to do errands. Having access to a bathroom is a priority, and when that access is uncertain, anxiety can result. It is understandable that most choose to take medications to help curb unpleasant symptoms, but long-term use of these can stress the body and cause other problems. A natural alternative is turmeric. This can be consumed to help alleviate the symptoms of ulcerative proctitis and colitis and may even keep the disease in remission.

Curcumin from turmeric was given to a small sample of patients with ulcerative proctitis. All patients improved their symptoms, and most were able to reduce the use of their medications.[84] In a larger six-month study, patients with inactive ulcerative colitis were given either a split dose of 2 grams of curcumin a day plus a commonly used anti-inflammatory or a placebo with the same anti-inflammatory. Patients treated with curcumin had significantly lower recurrence rates than those given placebos. Improvements were noted in the endoscopic index that measures vascular pattern, bleeding, and ulceration as well as in the clinical activity index that measures severity of symptoms.[85]

CHAPTER 2

ATTAIN PHYSICAL AND MENTAL WELLNESS

49. ALCOHOL INTOXICATION

Alcohol includes all forms of ethanol and is found in wine, champagne, beer, vodka, rum, whiskey, gin, tequila, brandy, cognac, and vermouth. It increases the effects of GABA, a neurotransmitter that sends messages to the brain and nervous system and slows down signals. Consuming excessive alcohol slows signals too much and leads to physical and mental impairment. These effects depend on health conditions, how frequently and how much the person drinks, the weight of the person, whether they are taking medications, or if they have food in their stomach. Twenty percent of alcohol is absorbed into the bloodstream directly from the stomach and 80 percent from the small intestine, and from there it is metabolized in the liver. After one drink, the person's skin may feel flushed and they may feel less inhibited. As more and more alcohol is consumed, slurring of speech, lack of judgment, poor coordination, emotional instability, and memory loss may be evident. Eventually the person may become stuporous or even comatose. Death is possible if blood pressure drops too low, breathing ceases, or vomit blocks the airways. Sobering up takes time. Cold showers and caffeine have a temporary effect and should not be relied upon to remove the symptoms of alcohol consumption.

Medications won't speed up the removal of alcohol from the body, but non-steroidal anti-inflammatories can help with the pain of a hangover. Curcumin can be used to reduce the extent of alcohol intoxication and subsequent hangovers. A branded form of microencapsulated nanoparticle curcumin with high absorption rates—twenty-seven times higher than curcumin powder—subdued drunkenness in humans as demonstrated by the reduction in blood concentration of acetaldehyde.[86] This compound is formed from the metabolism of alcohol in the liver, and higher amounts are found in the blood after drinking alcoholic beverages.

50. ANXIETY

Everyone feels anxiety at certain times in their life. Before going on a job interview, stepping out on a first date, or moving to a new city, you may experience fear, worry, nervousness, panic, or uneasiness. These feelings usually subside after the event has passed. For some, these feelings don't resolve and are persistent and overwhelming. This is another level of anxiety and is classified as an anxiety disorder. There are different types, but they can all interfere with normal life and be so intense and disabling that the afflicted withdraw from society. Anxiety is caused by changes in the function of the brain that regulates emotions. On a physiological level, the person may have shortness of breath, heart palpitations, nausea, muscle tension, and insomnia. Drugs can be used to reduce symptoms, counseling to address emotional issues, diet changes to improve overall body function, and relaxation techniques to self-soothe.

Some people with anxiety do require the help of doctors and counselors to assist them in dealing with psychological issues and physical symptoms. It does not matter if anxiety stems from normal fear and worry or from a diagnosed anxiety disorder. Taking oral doses of natural products like turmeric can also help. Curcumin extracts from turmeric were given over a twelve-week period to patients with depression. Not only was curcumin effective in reducing the symptoms of depression, but it was also active in reducing anxiety. The Spielberger State-Trait Anxiety Inventory scores, measuring the severity of anxiety symptoms in a self-reported manner, were improved after the use of curcumin.[87] Anxiety can be activated by chemicals like sulfite, a food preservative that can disturb the brain and induce anxiety. Curcumin had an anti-anxiety effect when fed to male rats exposed to sulfites.[88] On the other hand, the absence of a compound can also trigger anxiety as seen in the dietary deficiency of docosahexaenoic acid, DHA. Curcumin was able to enhance the synthesis of DHA, resulting in elevated levels in the brain and a reduction in the symptoms of anxiety.[89]

51. ARSENIC EXPOSURE

Arsenic is a semi-metallic chemical naturally found in minuscule amounts in the earth's crust. Some areas have higher amounts than others due to human activity such as pesticide use. It has become widely distributed in the water and air. Exposure in the United States is mainly through drinking contaminated water and through consuming food that had been irrigated with it or prepared in it. Antibiotics in chicken feed is another major source of exposure, as is some rice and tobacco. Worldwide, more than 200 million people are exposed to potentially unsafe levels of arsenic. Acute poisoning is followed by vomiting, diarrhea, abdominal pain, tingling in the extremities, and sometimes death. Long-term exposure is associated with skin lesions and skin cancer, cardiovascular disease, diabetes, and neurotoxicity leading to physical and cognitive impairment. Treatment for arsenic poisoning is designed to remove arsenic from the body and minimize damage. Sometimes blood transfusions are necessary. Bowel irrigation and chelation therapy can remove traces of arsenic. Mineral supplements or medications can be used to protect organs from damage.

The ubiquitous nature of arsenic makes avoiding exposure nearly impossible. Most people will inhale or ingest traces of arsenic throughout their lives. It seems prudent to actively protect the body from arsenic poisoning. A safe and natural way to do this is to consume curcumin from turmeric. Blood samples of people in regions of West Bengal where high levels of arsenic poisoning are common found severe DNA damage and increased oxidative stress. After three months of curcumin use, DNA damage was reduced. Antioxidant activity increased, and the levels of reactive oxygen species decreased, providing this protective effect.[90] Daily curcumin consumption can safeguard against DNA damage and further health complications from chronic arsenic exposure.

52. BABY ROoT CANAL

If a cavity in a child's baby tooth is deep enough, it may reach the nerve or pulp of the tooth. Bacteria can enter deep into the tooth and begin an infection. If left unattended, the infection can spread to the bloodstream and cause a number of medical conditions.

To avoid this, a baby root canal is recommended to save the tooth and prevent bacterial buildup. All the pulp tissue of the tooth is removed and replaced with a sterile filling and sealing material. These medications can move into the bloodstream as well and cause unintended harm throughout the body. The importance of finding phytochemical fillers and sealers with inherent antibacterial activity and a high safety profile is warranted. It may seem unnecessary to save a baby tooth, but they are essential to speech development and to maintain alignment for the permanent teeth.

As an alternative, turmeric powder mixed with distilled water and radiolucent material was used to replace infected pulp in children's teeth. After six months, 93 percent of patients reported no pain, and none of them felt any tenderness or fistula—symptoms that would indicate infection. The anti-inflammatory and antibacterial properties of turmeric appear to be effective in safely restoring the health to previously infected baby teeth.[91]

53. BLOOD THINNER

Blood clots are necessary to stop bleeding, but they can also form in places in the body where they can be dangerous. In the arteries and veins, blood clots can form in an attempt to repair tissue damage by laying down layers of fibrin and platelets. This is a problem because these clots slow the flow of blood. They can block blood vessels completely at their site of origin, or they can break off and plug a vein or artery elsewhere in the body. This can be extremely serious and lead to heart attack or stroke. Depending on where the clot is located, treatment can be with either anticoagulation medications or with acetaminophen or ibuprofen to manage pain and inflammation. Some side effects of anticoagulants include severe bruising, bleeding gums, vomiting blood, chest pain, and prolonged nose bleeds.

Curcumin is proposed as an anticoagulant to prevent the formation of blood clots in at-risk patients, without the side effects of traditional anticoagulant drugs. It increases the production of prostacyclin, a powerful inhibitor of platelet aggregation. Interestingly, acetylsalicylic acid, which is commonly taken to thin the blood, inhibited its production.[92] Curcumin, in a bioavailable form, is likely a more effective blood thinner than aspirin.

54. COGNITIVE FUNCTION

The attainment and processing of knowledge is a direct function of cognition-mental processes that include perception, memory, reasoning, judgment, attention, and language. Each person is unique and will differ in how they see and react to the world around them. Genetics accounts for the majority of cognitive variation seen in the general population. Environmental factors and physiological processes make up the rest. Chemical imbalances and changes in metabolic pathways can bring a noticeable change in cognition over time. Some of these processes can be triggered with age, dietary deficiencies, or exogenous chemical or pathogen exposure. Memory and thinking skills can become impaired.

A twelve-month study in older adults investigated the effect of consuming a highly bioavailable form of curcumin on preventing cognitive decline. Curcumin successfully prevented loss of function, while the opposite effect was noted in the placebo group of adults.[93] Curcumin also elevates docosahexaenoic acid levels in the brain, a deficiency of which is linked to several cognitive disorders.[94] Taking curcumin on a daily basis is an effective way to prevent cognitive impairment and even reverse it in certain cases.

HEALTH

WELLNESS

BEAUTY

CRAFTS

HEALTH

WELLNESS

BEAUTY

CRAFTS

55. COLD SORES

Cold sores, or fever blisters, are herpes simplex viral (HSV-1) infections that affect the skin around the mouth. Fluid-filled sores develop in and around the lips, eventually breaking and leaking a clear liquid. A crust then forms. Cold sores tend to group in clusters and are red, swollen, and sore and can be accompanied by fever and swollen neck glands. Some cold sores only last a few days, while others take weeks to go away. The herpes simplex virus is contagious, and touching the area or sharing utensils, toothbrushes, or razors can spread the infection. The virus gets into the skin through any scratch or tiny cut, so if an outbreak is underway, don't kiss anyone goodnight or share a glass of wine! Once the virus is contracted, it will always be there. It is not always known why an outbreak occurs, but stress and a depressed immune system are thought to be triggers. Antiviral creams, ointments, or pills can reduce symptoms but usually only get rid of the cold sores one or two days quicker than without treatment.

Those few days, however, can be extremely important to people during an outbreak. The sores cause not only pain but embarrassment for some. The initial tingling sensation associated with an impending outbreak can have a person running for medication or even hiding out until the cold sores have cleared up.

A major problem with current antiviral drugs is drug resistance. Finding a natural antiviral, especially one commonly found in the home, provides a new and accessible agent to fight the herpes simplex virus. In laboratory experiments, curcumin and two of its

derivatives were found to be very effective in preventing the replication of cold sore–forming herpes simplex virus cells.[95]

At the first sign of a cold sore, mix 1/4 teaspoon of raw honey
with 1/8 teaspoon of ground turmeric. Make a paste and apply to
the area. Leave on for thirty minutes. Rinse off. Do this several
times a day. The paste will hasten the healing process but should
also reduce pain and itching.

56. COMMON COLD

The common cold is a respiratory illness that can be caused by
many different viruses. They are highly contagious, and a person
can become infected by touching a surface such as a doorknob,
stair railing, or bathroom faucet. If the virus gets on the hands and
the person then touches their mouth or nose, the virus nestles into
the mucosal lining there. Breathing in air near someone who is
coughing or sneezing because they are sick with a cold is another
surefire way of getting the virus into the system. Unless the body
has fought the exact virus before, it won't have the right antibodies
ready to fight it when it enters the body. The immune system begins
an attack against the new virus, and the dreaded symptoms set in.
A sore throat, runny or stuffy nose, sneezing, and cough are the
hallmarks of a cold. There is no shortage of over-the-counter cold
medications, and they are available for every possible symptom.
Take a walk down the pharmacy aisle to see antihistamines, decongestants, nasal sprays, cough suppressants, and throat lozenges.

The respiratory syncytial virus is one of the most common
viruses causing cold symptoms. Silver nanoparticles modified

by the addition of curcumin were highly effective at inhibiting respiratory syncytial viral infections by directly inactivating the virus.[96] When curcumin was combined with lactoferrin, a protein with antiviral activity, and supplemented to healthy children with recurrent respiratory tract infections, the number of infections was reduced.[97] To beat a cold, try this drink.

HOT TURMERIC MILK

1 teaspoon raw honey
1/2 teaspoon ground turmeric
1/4 teaspoon ground ginger
1/4 teaspoon cinnamon
pinch of black pepper
1 cup milk or non-dairy alternative

Mix ingredients in a pan and heat on the stove over medium heat, stirring constantly until warmed.

57. DEPRESSION

Depression is a mood disorder that causes a deep sadness and a loss of interest in activities. It affects how a person feels, thinks, and behaves and can cause not just emotional problems but physical problems as well. Clinical depression may occur once in a person's lifetime or reoccur multiple times. This feeling of sadness and loss can cause insomnia, loss of appetite, poor concentration, fatigue, suicidal thoughts, and physical symptoms like backaches and headaches. Changes in the body's hormone levels may cause or trigger depression. Modifications of the way brain chemicals work and the effect that has on maintaining stable moods is thought to play a major role. Psychological counseling and antidepressant medications are often prescribed. Antidepressants can cause a wide range of side effects, including nausea, insomnia, blurred vision, weight gain, fatigue, and sexual dysfunction.

Curcumin appears to be safe, effective, and well tolerated among patients diagnosed with depressive disorders. In mice models, curcumin increased the levels of serotonin, noradrenaline, and dopamine neurotransmitters in the brain that may play a role in alleviating depression.[98] In human trials, curcumin alone and in combination with saffron significantly reduced depressive symptoms in patients with major depressive disorders.[99] Its efficacy was not dose dependent. Another trial showed it was even comparable to fluoxetine, a common drug prescribed to treat depression. Curcumin was well tolerated by all the patients and showed no adverse symptoms, unlike fluoxetine.[100]

58. DIARRHEA

The term *diarrhea* describes loose, watery stools. It is a very common condition and usually lasts a few days, although prolonged diarrhea can indicate a medical condition like irritable bowel syndrome. Stomach cramps and pain, bloating, fever, nausea, and vomiting often accompany diarrhea. It occurs when the stool moves too quickly through the colon, so the colon doesn't have time to absorb enough liquid from it. The main culprits in causing diarrhea are viruses, bacteria, and parasites. Food intolerance and many medications can also cause diarrhea in susceptible people. If diarrhea persists for more than a few days, doctors may prescribe antibiotics if the cause is bacterial or parasitic.

Increased resistance to antibiotics is a major problem in treating infectious bacterial diseases. Alternative therapies need to be developed to be used in place of, or in combination with, current treatments to provide relief in resistant cases. Curcumin used in combination with three antibiotics was tested against five strains of bacteria causing diarrhea. Curcumin was able to reduce the dose of antibiotics used while still remaining as effective as the original higher dose without curcumin. It even had a synergistic effect with one of the antibiotics, making treatment more effective than before.[101]

59. DRY EYES

Tears are needed to ensure the health and comfort of our eyes. There are three layers to tears: An outer oily layer keeps tears from drying up too quickly. A watery middle layer cleans the eye by washing away particles and grit. A mucus inner layer helps spread the watery layer over the eye to keep it moist. If production of one or more of these layers is diminished, dry eye can result. This is a very common condition that affects millions of Americans and is more prevalent in women than men. Not only is it uncomfortable, it is downright irritating. The eyes can burn, itch, ache, or feel heavy and tired. They may be red and inflamed or sensitive to light. Wearing contacts can become painful. The overproduction of mucus or water may result as the eye's way of overcompensating, but this doesn't correct the underlying dry eye condition. The use of artificial tears can be helpful. If these drops are used frequently, be sure to purchase preservative-free brands so the chemicals in them don't irritate your eyes. Another option is to have an ophthalmologist insert a tiny device into the tear duct to block drainage and increase the eye's surface moisture.

Dry eyes have less water and more salt than normal tears. This increase in salt concentration causes inflammation in the eye. In a dry eye model using corneal epithelial cells, pretreatment with curcumin was able to inhibit the production of compounds that promote inflammation. The corneal epithelial cells themselves were not damaged.[102] This suggests that turmeric or curcumin supplementation may have potential in reducing the inflammatory symptom of dry eyes.

60. ECZEMA

This is a group of medical conditions that cause the skin to become itchy and inflamed. It is often accompanied by asthma or hay fever and is common in infants, affecting up to 20 percent, although most outgrow eczema by their tenth birthday. It also affects about 3 percent of children and adults, who experience it on and off throughout their lives. During a flare-up, the skin is itchy, thickened, dry, and scaly. The skin may be red or brown, and pigmentation could be affected. There are many triggers that cause flare-ups, including scratching, hot showers, stress, clothing, or allergens. Nearly all people with eczema have *Staphylococcus aureus* bacteria on the skin, which multiply rapidly if they penetrate the surface. If this happens, symptoms worsen. Creams and oral drugs to control itching and inflammation can help manage symptoms, and antibiotics can help clear up an infection.

HEALTH

WELLNESS

BEAUTY

CRAFTS

The main goal for treatment of eczema is to relieve itching, since scratching can lead to infection. Curcumin in turmeric decreases scratching behavior in mice[103] and decreases the severity of itching in humans, in part by lowering the release of pro-inflammatory proteins from the liver.[104] Curcumin's anti-inflammatory activity can help reduce swelling and redness of affected tissue. Another compound found in turmeric, called hydroxycinnamic acid, inhibits the activation of T cells and the production of proteins needed for the inflammatory response.[105] This may decrease the incidence of flare-ups and make the body's response more moderate. If *Staphylococcus aureus* causes a skin infection, curcumin can destroy these bacteria by damaging their membranes, allowing contents to leak out.[106] Taking turmeric orally or using it topically on the skin shows therapeutic potential in the treatment of eczema.

61. EYE INFLAMMATION

Swelling of eye tissue can result from infections, trauma, or auto-immune disorders or be part of inflammatory diseases originating in other parts of the body. It can happen at any age but primarily hits between the ages of twenty and sixty years. Some cases are acute and resolve quickly, while others are chronic and can last for a long time, with multiple recurrences. Vision is diminished, and the patients often complain of floaters. These are often white blood cells that have leaked out of the blood vessels in the eye. Blurred vision, redness, and light sensitivity are also common. Steroidal anti-inflammatory medications are prescribed to reduce swelling, pain, and further tissue damage. Some side effects of these are osteoporosis, ulcers, glaucoma, cataracts, and cardiovascular insults.

The seriousness of the potential side effects of steroid use requires safer methods to treat inflammation of the eye. Curcumin (375 milligrams, three times a day) given orally for twelve weeks to patients suffering from chronic inflammation of the anterior part of the eye showed improvements in their condition and a lower recurrence rate. The results were comparable to corticosteroid therapy, but no side effects were reported.[107] Daily consumption of turmeric or curcumin supplements may be effective enough to reduce or replace steroid use in patients.

62. FLU

Seasonal flu is a respiratory illness caused by influenza A and B viruses. The viruses are contagious, and a person can become infected by touching a surface with the virus and transferring it to the mouth or nose. Here, the virus nestles into the mucosal lining and begins to replicate. Contaminated people who cough or sneeze cause the virus to become airborne. Simply breathing in this air can begin an infection. Symptoms can be mild or severe and, in certain cases, fatal. Symptoms include a fever, sore throat, runny or stuffy nose, cough, fatigue, muscle aches, and headaches. At its onset, antiviral drugs can be taken to shorten the duration of the illness by one or two days and lessen the severity of symptoms.

Each year, many people opt to get a flu vaccine to prevent seasonal influenza. This is not a guarantee that you won't get sick, however. If you do get sick and don't want to take antiviral drugs because of the possible side effects (including nausea, vomiting, diarrhea, and headaches), then taking curcumin may be your answer to feeling better sooner. Human and mice immune cells infected with influenza A viruses and subsequently treated with curcumin decreased the inflammatory response.[108] This would lead to a milder form of infection with fewer and less severe symptoms. Curcumin also acts to inhibit the viral infection by disrupting the integrity of the viral membrane, causing its contents to leak.[109] This prevents the virus from replicating and spreading throughout the body, limiting its reach and ending the infection sooner.

63. HEART PROTECTION

Reactive oxygen species (ROS) are reactive molecules and free radicals derived from oxygen that are produced as byproducts of chemical processes in the body. ROS are very destructive to cells and are implicated in aging, chronic disease, and cancer. When levels of ROS prove too high for existing antioxidants to handle, the body is under oxidative stress. The heart muscle is not immune to the destructive nature of ROS; ROS can cause changes in the size, shape, structure, and function of this organ and even lead to heart failure. Environmental stressors like pollutants, tobacco, smoke, radiation, and drugs can increase ROS levels.

The body defends against ROS through the work of antioxidants. They scavenge the ROS and make them stable so they no longer cause damage. When increased ROS levels are present, more antioxidants are needed to quell them. If the body has a high enough reserve, homeostasis can be achieved. However, sometimes additional antioxidants are needed to reach this balance and prevent the body from entering a state of oxidative stress. Curcumin is an antioxidant and has potential as a therapeutic agent in preventing damage to the heart muscle induced by ROS. This type of damage is often generated by adriamycin, a drug used in cancer treatment. Adriamycin elevates levels of ROS, which attack heart muscle tissue and cause cardiotoxicity. Curcumin treatment seven days before and two days after injection of rats with Adriamycin significantly reduced damage to the heart muscle.[110] Curcumin can be taken to increase existing antioxidant levels in the body and provide a protective effect not only to the heart but to other tissues in the body as well. It can also be taken along with adriamycin to limit ROS damage to the heart during cancer treatment. Make sure to check with your doctor before adding a curcumin supplement in this case.

64. INDIGESTION

An *upset stomach* is a general term that describes a number of symptoms like bloating, heartburn, burping, nausea, or pain the upper middle part of the stomach. These symptoms are often brought on by acid reflux, a digestive disease in which the muscle between the stomach and esophagus does not close properly and stomach acid moves up into the esophagus. This damages the protective lining of the esophagus, causing inflammation and irritation. Stomach ulcers, anti-inflammatory medications, and infections are other causes. Infections are treated with antibiotics, while acid reflux is reduced with antacids, H-2-receptor antagonists, and proton pump inhibitors. Prokinetics can be administered to speed up the emptying of the stomach. Changes in diet may also help, as can the cessation of smoking.

The medications primarily used for the treatment of indigestion can bring a slew of other complaints. They include diarrhea, constipation, headaches, nausea, vomiting, back pain, abdominal pain (which seems counterintuitive), flatulence, anxiety, and depression. An alternative option with far fewer and less serious side effects is to use plant extracts. A commercial mixture of various plants including turmeric was used to treat patients with indigestion from unknown causes. After sixty days, a significant reduction of symptom severity was recorded, with 79 percent of these patients having at least half of their symptoms improved.[111] Another trial carried out among six hospitals gave patients with indigestion turmeric capsules or placebo capsules for seven days. Eighty-seven percent of patients taking turmeric responded positively to the treatment.[112] Side effects were mild and self-limiting.

65. IRRITABLE BOWEL SYNDROME

Irritable bowel syndrome (IBS) is a common intestinal disorder of the colon. It occurs when the muscles in the intestines contract more strongly or for longer periods of time than normal, or the contractions may be weak and slow the progression of food through the body. Abnormalities in the nervous system in the colon may also be responsible. IBS doesn't cause changes in the bowel tissue, however, and does not increase the risk of cancer like the inflammatory bowel diseases, Crohn's, and ulcerative colitis. It does, however, affect quality of life because the onset of symptoms can be unpredictable and come at inconvenient times, causing stress for the sufferer.

Abdominal pain and cramps are often the first signs that the bowel is acting up. Diarrhea or constipation commonly follow with the expulsion of excessive gas and sometimes mucus in the stool. It is not uncommon to experience alternating episodes of diarrhea and constipation. IBS is chronic and cannot be cured, but symptoms often go away for periods of time, affording the person some relief. It is not known what causes irritable bowel, but each person has their own set of triggers that can cause symptoms to appear. Common triggers are particular foods, stress, hormones, and other gastrointestinal illnesses. Because the cause of IBS is unknown, changes in lifestyle are recommended to manage the condition. Learning to avoid any food triggers, decreasing stress, and taking probiotics are recommended. Doctor-prescribed medicines like antispasmodics, antidepressants, and antibiotics can treat IBS symptoms but may cause other gastrointestinal upsets, weight gain, fatigue, blurred vision, headaches, and more.

Taking turmeric each day can help with the uncomfortable and sometimes painful symptoms associated with irritable bowel syndrome. Standardized turmeric extracts taken daily for eight weeks resulted in a significant decrease of symptoms with approximately two-thirds of patients reporting better bowel function.[113] This is a simple and cost-effective alternative to prescription drugs and has little to no side effects.

66. LIVER PROTECTION

The liver is the largest internal organ in the body. It filters toxins out of the bloodstream to prevent them from damaging tissues. When the liver tissue itself becomes damaged, it has the ability to regenerate and make new, healthy tissue. When the damage gets too extensive, however, liver disease sets in, and it no longer functions as it should. A number of conditions can cause liver disease, including hepatitis A, B, and C; cirrhosis of the liver; nonalcoholic fatty liver disease; and alcoholic hepatitis. Poisons, medications, and viruses are other causes. Symptoms include abdominal swelling and pain, bruising, fatigue, loss of appetite, and jaundice.

The liver is constantly bombarded with hazardous compounds that threaten the health of various tissues in the body or the individual as a whole. If not metabolized into harmless compounds or excreted out of the body, these compounds become toxic to the liver and impair its critical functions. It is imperative that the liver be protected so that it continues to defend the rest of the body. Curcumin has been found to provide this protection as demonstrated in a number of liver toxicity studies. Drugs taken during tuberculosis treatment are linked to liver damage in up to 11 percent of patients.[114] Curcumin and another plant extract, *Tinospora cordifolia*, were used in combination with conventional treatment in tuberculosis-positive patients. These herbs were able to significantly prevent liver damage induced by the treatment drugs, without any side effects.[115] The effect of other liver-damaging compounds was also significantly attenuated by the administration of curcumin. The poison thallium acetate,[116] iron,[117] alcohol, and oxidized oil[118] were all studied for their effect in rat livers. Curcumin reduced oxidative stress and attenuated negative impacts on biochemical processes induced by each of these compounds. It appears that taking a daily prophylactic (preventative) dose of curcumin would provide protection against toxic environmental and food compounds constantly harming the liver.

67. MIGRAINE

Migraines are severe headaches that cause intense pain, usually on one side of the head, and are accompanied by nausea, vomiting, and sensitivity to light and sound. Migraines can come with warning signs such as blind spots in the field of vision, flashes of light, or tingling sensations on the face, arms, or legs. Migraines can be so severe that the person can't function normally and often requires rest and isolation to recover. Causes of migraines are different for everyone. Some triggers could be changes in hormone levels, food allergies, stress, some medications, sensory stimuli, or changes in the environment, like a fall in barometric pressure from an approaching storm. They may also be symptoms of disease. Pain-relieving and anti-nausea medications are commonly used to deal with the symptoms.

Tumor necrosis factor (TNF)-α is an inflammatory protein that appears to play a role in the development of migraines. A nano-formulation of curcumin combined with omega-3 fatty acids administered to migraine patients over a two-month period significantly decreased the serum levels of (TNF)-α in a synergistic manner. This resulted in a greatly reduced frequency of migraine attacks in patients taking both nano-curcumin and omega-3 fatty acids.[119] Supplementing with both these compounds could provide relief to many sufferers to help alleviate inflammation and pain and reduce the number of recurrent episodes.

68. MUSCLE PAIN

After months of inactivity, going out for a competitive game of flag football or a vigorous evening run with a friend may seem like a good idea. However, trying to move about the next day when every muscle is stiff and sore will squelch that belief. Taking preventative measures to guard against injury-induced muscle pain or aches from overuse are something to think about for next time. Muscle aches can also result from tension, stress, or disease. The pain can be anywhere in the body and last from several hours to months. If exercise induced, muscle pain results from microscopic tears in the muscle fibers, while if disease related, it can be caused by inflammation.

Oral curcumin supplementation can decrease the delayed onset of muscle soreness that is common after intense workouts or when working new muscle groups. Seventeen men were given either 2.5 grams of curcumin or placebo twice a day beginning two days before exercise and continuing for three days after. After one and two days, moderate to large reductions in pain were noted by participants during single leg squats, squat jumps, and gluteal stretches. There was also a small increase in exercise performance in the single leg jump.[120] Curcumin can be taken to minimize muscle pain and may even improve performance in subsequent workouts.

69. NEUROPATHIC PAIN, AS A COMPLICATION OF DIABETES

The most chronic complication of diabetes is neuropathy, damage of the nerves throughout the body. There are four types: Peripheral neuropathy is the most common and causes tingling, burning, stabbing, or sharp shooting pains in the feet, legs, hands, and arms. Pain may be worse at night. Up to 50 percent of people with peripheral neuropathy experience no pain. Often their extremities go numb, increasing the risk of foot ulcers and amputations. Autonomic neuropathy affects the nerves that control the heart, digestive system, sex organs, sweat glands, and bladder and can create issues associated with the functioning of all these organs. Proximal neuropathy weakens nerves in the thighs, hips, buttocks, and legs. Sudden, severe pain or trouble standing up are indicators. Mononeuropathy targets just one nerve.

Diabetic neuropathy is related to high blood sugar and tends to worsen with age and duration since onset. High blood pressure, obesity, high cholesterol, high triglycerides, and smoking are other contributing factors. The best way to manage diabetic nerve pain is to keep blood sugar levels under tight control. Medications to manage pain can be used, but they don't work for everyone and have many side effects.

This condition is difficult to treat, and the amount of relief pain medications provide often doesn't justify the additional health issues that arise with their use. Chronic curcumin treatment in diabetic mice significantly lowered sensitivity to pain, possibly by inhibiting the release of factors involved in systemic inflammation and in the transmission of nerve pain signals.[121] Curcumin can also help slow the progression of neuropathy through its ability to control blood sugar levels. It modulates these levels in diabetic patients[122] and increases insulin secretion.[123] Turmeric, specifically curcumin, is a promising alternative to the chronic use of prescription medications to control nerve pain.

70. ORAL LICHEN PLANUS

This is an allergic reaction that affects the mouth, although it can also affect the skin, esophagus, and vaginal mucosa. It is relatively common, found in about 2 percent of the population, but appears most commonly in women over fifty. It can look like a white, lacy, thread-like pattern. This mild form is found mostly on the cheeks and doesn't usually require treatment. Another form appears as bright red and inflamed tissue on the gums, tongue, and cheeks. The top layer of mucosa is lost, resulting in pain while eating and drinking. Ulcers can form in severe cases, causing chronic pain and discomfort. Topical corticosteroids are used to reduce inflammation and maintain control over the symptoms of the disease.

One of the corticosteroids used to treat oral lichen planus is triamcinolone acetonide. It lessens inflammation and redness of the oral cavity and can be useful in reducing the discomfort of mouth sores. This corticosteroid was given to one group of patients diagnosed with oral lichen planus. Curcumin oral gel was given to two other comparable groups in either a low or high dose over three months. All three groups showed significant reduction in the redness of oral tissue and in ulceration. Burning sensation, another common symptom, was also reduced. Triamcinolone acetonide was the most effective, followed by the higher dose of curcumin oral gel. The authors advise using a course of corticosteroids to get the condition under control then switching to curcumin to maintain oral lichen planus in a remissive state.[124]

71. OSTEOPENIA

Osteopenia is often confused with osteoporosis. Both involve lower-than normal levels of bone density, but osteopenia is less serious.

Bones contain minerals that make them strong and dense. The body is constantly breaking down and reabsorbing old bone cells and making new bone cells using calcium. Peak bone density is reached around thirty years of age. After this, the process of bone-cell reabsorption gradually outpaces bone-cell formation, and bone density decreases. This makes the bones weaker and susceptible to fracture. Loss of estrogen during menopause, diets deficient in calcium and vitamin D, smoking, alcohol abuse, and some medications and medical conditions are risk factors that can contribute to the development of osteopenia. This condition is more prevalent in women because they have smaller and thinner bones than men. Often, people don't know they have it until they have a bone density test.

HEALTH

WELLNESS

BEAUTY

CRAFTS

It's important to keep bones strong in an effort to prevent low bone mass, a precursor to osteoporosis. In addition to dietary and lifestyle changes as well as regular weight-bearing exercise, taking curcumin may help slow the progression of bone loss. Healthy subjects with low bone density were given an oral-based curcumin supplement. A control group not supplemented with curcumin was used for comparison. After twenty-four weeks, bone densities measured in the heel, small finger, and upper jaw were significantly increased in the curcumin-supplemented group, while no such changes were observed in the control group.[125]

72. PREMENSTRUAL SYNDRoME

Women of child-bearing years often experience pain and cramping just before or during the first few days of menstruation. Pain can be mild to severe and is described as a dull, throbbing ache in the lower abdomen, hips, back, and thighs. It usually lasts twelve to seventy-two hours and, for some, can prevent normal activities for several days. It happens when the muscles of the woman's uterus contract too strongly and put pressure on nearby blood vessels. The oxygen supply to muscle tissue of the uterus is temporarily cut off, and pain results. Over-the-counter pain relievers and hormone birth control are used to relieve pain. Primary menstrual cramps usually occur each menstrual cycle and can be associated with other symptoms like nausea, vomiting, diarrhea, and fatigue. They are differentiated from secondary menstrual pain, which has an underlying cause like a reproductive disorder or infection.

The main objective in managing this condition is to reduce pain and treat the symptoms.

Curcumin is able to do just this. A study of healthy women with premenstrual syndrome were divided into two groups. The first received 100 milligrams of curcumin every twelve hours beginning seven days before the onset of menstrual bleeding and continuing for three days after. The second group received placebos over the same timeline. Women in the curcumin group reported significant improvements in their physical, behavioral, and mood premenstrual symptoms compared to their symptoms before the trial. Women in the placebo group did not report such improvements.[126] It is speculated that curcumin's effects were attributed to its ability to reduce inflammation and pain as well as modulate neurotransmitter activity, resulting in elevated mood.

73. PSORIASIS

Psoriasis is a common skin condition caused when skin cells grow ten times faster than normal. This overabundance of cells creates raised red plaques with silvery scales on the surface of the skin. These patches can be itchy and painful, and the skin can dry, crack, and bleed. Nails can also become pitted and discolored. Up to 30 percent of people with psoriasis also have psoriatic arthritis and experience pain and swelling in their joints. Most cases of psoriasis go through periods of flare-up and remission and can be triggered by stress, certain medications, infection, skin injury, smoking, or cold weather. These triggers send a faulty immune system into action. Some of the body's white blood cells attack healthy skin cells, provoking other immune responses that cause

HEALTH

WELLNESS

BEAUTY

CRAFTS

the proliferation of skin cells, redness, inflammation, and other symptoms. There is no cure, but psoriasis can be managed with topical treatments, light therapy, and oral or injectable drugs.

To date, the best that can be hoped for in those with psoriasis is to keep the condition in remission as long as possible and to treat the symptoms of flare-up as they occur.

Topical medication in combination with ultraviolet A (UVA) radiation is the preferred treatment for extensive moderate-to-severe plaque psoriasis. However, orally administered curcumin shows similar therapeutic potential when combined with visible light phototherapy. The combination of curcumin and UVA radiation was also effective at reducing the body surface area affected by psoriasis after treatment, but slightly less so than curcumin and visible light.[127] The importance of this is that using visible light phototherapy is much less harmful to the body than UVA radiation, providing a safer treatment than current methods.

74. SPRAINS

Ligaments are fibrous tissue that attach bone to bone. Tearing or overextending a ligament can result in a sprain. Pain, swelling, bruising, and limited movement are felt in the area of the injury. Sprains happen most often in the ankle from walking or running on uneven surfaces. The knee, wrist, and thumb are other common sites of injury. Making sure to warm up properly before exercising, stopping when muscles are fatigued, wearing proper footwear, and avoiding slippery or uneven surfaces can reduce your risk of a sprain. Proper physical conditioning is also helpful to avoid injury from playing sports. Most minor sprains can be treated at home.

Rest the area, apply ice for twenty minutes, and repeat every few hours; compress the area with an elastic bandage and elevate the injury. This should reduce swelling. Pain can be managed with over-the-counter medications like ibuprofen and acetaminophen. More severe sprains may require the attention of a doctor and physical therapist.

Reducing swelling will help alleviate pain and provide relief to the injured person. Both oral ingestion and topical application of curcumin is useful in this regard.

TURMERIC PASTE FOR SPRAINS

1. Mix two parts ground turmeric with one part salt, and add just enough water to make a paste. Spread the paste over the sprained tissue and wrap it in a cloth.
2. Bear in mind that the cloth will stain permanently and the skin temporarily. To remove the yellow color from skin, simply rub a cotton ball dipped in coconut oil over the skin.

Ground turmeric can be eaten as part of the diet, thrown in stir-frys, curries, hot milk, or tea, or taken as a capsule. Turmeric taken alongside bromelain, another anti-inflammatory compound, has a synergistic effect and works well to reduce swelling from sprains. Take these two to three times a day, or as directed, to help recover from injury.

75. TOOTHACHE

Pain in or around a tooth that is sharp or throbbing is a toothache. The pain may be constant or only when pressure is applied to the tooth and is generally a result of the tooth's nerve root becoming irritated. Swelling around the tooth and headaches sometimes occur. Some causes are tooth decay, damaged fillings, infected gums, trauma to the tooth, or teeth grinding. Dental treatment is often necessary to fix a damaged tooth. Over-the-counter pain medications are used to temporarily dull pain and inflammation.

An alternative to these medications, like ibuprofen or acetaminophen, is turmeric. This is an anti-inflammatory that can reduce swelling in the mouth and, subsequently, pain. (See Turmeric Mouthwash, page 33.)

76. WEIGHT LOSS

Having too much body fat increases the risk of health problems like diabetes, heart disease, and certain cancers. Losing weight can improve or prevent any weight-induced conditions. Fat accumulates on the body when more calories are eaten than burned. The body stores these excess calories as fat. Exercising and eating a healthy diet with appropriate calorie intake will help burn the stored fat and reduce body weight.

Metabolic processes that occur during increasing fat-tissue deposition in the body lead to chronic low-grade inflammation. The anti-inflammatory compound curcumin can encourage weight loss by directly interacting with white fat tissue, the type of tissue that stores excess fat. It promotes the expression of an anti-inflammatory protein, causing a suppression of inflammation. It also acts to restrict the development of new fat cells.[128] In a trial of overweight subjects, curcumin administered for thirty days resulted in an increase in weight loss, body fat reduction, and a reduction in waistline, hip circumference, and body mass index.[129] It even appears to protect against weight regain following cessation of diet and exercise.[130] The high tolerability and lack of side effects makes curcumin a potential weight loss management candidate that can be used in place of other supplements known to have unpleasant side effects.

77. WEST NILE PREVENTION

West Nile virus (WNV) is spread from its natural host, birds, to mosquitos and then to humans. When mosquitos feed on infected birds, the virus makes its way from the blood to the salivary glands of the mosquito, where it can easily be injected into humans during a blood meal. This is the most common form of transmission, but organ transplants, blood transfusions, and breast milk are other ways this virus has spread in humans. About 80 percent of those infected with WNV do not exhibit any symptoms. The remaining 20 percent often get headaches, fever, fatigue, body aches, nausea, and vomiting. These symptoms are sometimes accompanied by a body rash and swollen lymph glands. A small proportion of the infected develop a more serious infection that affects the neurological system and can lead to paralysis. Treatment in symptomatic patients involves supportive care at home or in a hospital. *Culex quinquefasciatus* is the particular mosquito that carries this virus and is a widespread sub-tropical species found worldwide, including the southern United States.

No vaccines or specific antiviral treatments are currently available for WNV. The best practice is to prevent being bitten by mosquitos to avoid transmission of the virus. While it may not be feasible to stay indoors during mosquito season, applying an effective mosquito repellent specific to *Culex quinquefasciatus* would certainly help. Turmeric oil with vanillin repelled *Culex quinquefasciatus* for up to 8 hours and was similar in protection to the commonly used repellent DEET.[131]

When going outside, apply turmeric oil and vanillin in a carrier oil (2 drops each in 1 teaspoon of oil) to exposed skin to protect against mosquito bites. Turmeric is also effective at killing *Culex quinquefasciatus* mosquito larvae. It can be added to a mosquito control program to keep populations low. Very low concentrations are needed, and non-target organisms were not harmed.[132]

78. WOUND HEALING

Skin wounds happens to everyone. Whether it's slicing the tip of the finger while dicing carrots or slipping on gravel and scraping a knee, cuts and scrapes tear the skin tissue and often cause bleeding.

If the wound is deep, bleeds heavily, or has an object embedded in it, seek medical attention. If it's minor, however, it can be addressed at home. Wash your hands with soap and water. Clean the cut or scrape by pouring cool, clean water over it to remove dirt and debris. Then wash with soap and water. Once clean, an antibiotic ointment can be applied.

Curcumin is known to have significant wound-healing properties. As an antioxidant, it reduces the immune system's inflammatory response and decreases swelling and pain. It also enhances the rate at which new tissue is developed to close the wound. A study used an enhanced skin-delivery curcumin formulation, which was applied over wounds on rats once a day. After fourteen days, significant improvements in wound healing were noted. New skin cells grew, new blood vessels were formed, collagen was synthesized, and new connective tissue was created. These fill the wound with healthy, viable tissue. The growth of bacteria was also inhibited, compared to controls.[133] These results occur in both normal wounded tissue and in slow-healing tissue, as is often the case in diabetics. Both oral and topical application of curcumin appear to be effective in speeding wound repair.[134]

TURMERIC PASTE FOR SUPERFICIAL WOUNDS

1 teaspoon coconut oil
1/4 teaspoon ground turmeric root

1. Mix the two ingredients together and spread evenly over the wound.
2. Cover with a bandage to prevent the mixture from staining clothes.

79. ZIKA PREVENTION

The *Aedes* mosquito carries the Zika virus, the same mosquito that spreads dengue and yellow fever. They live indoors and outdoors and usually bite people during the day but are still active at night. The bite of an infected mosquito transfers the Zika virus to the person, who may then experience mild symptoms of fever, rash, joint pain, muscle pain, headache, and red eyes for several days. This virus can be transmitted through sexual contact and from mother to child during pregnancy. It is dangerous to the developing fetus and can cause severe brain defects, including microcephaly. Because this illness is usually mild (except in developing babies), no specific treatment is required. Rest, fluids, and over-the-counter pain and fever medications are recommended.

Reducing or eliminating mosquito populations in the area are important to lower the risk of being bitten. Empty standing water and other mosquito breeding sites. Wear protective clothing when outdoors, covering as much of the body as possible. Use insect repellent and keep doors and windows closed if no screens are in place. The World Health Organization recommends using insect repellent containing DEET or IR3535. While effective, DEET and IR3535 can be very irritating to the eyes. Both are able to dissolve plastics.

A natural alternative to use is turmeric. The essential oil from turmeric combined with vanillin was able to repel *Aedes aegypti* mosquitos for 150 minutes.[135] When different areas of the turmeric plant were investigated, the essential oils from the leaf and rhizome, as well as an ethanolic extract of the rhizome, showed *Aedes aegypti* mosquito biting deterrence similar to DEET. The pure compound ar-turmerone found in turmeric actually showed higher efficacy than DEET in preventing mosquito bites.[136] These oils can be combined with vanillin and a carrier oil and used directly on the skin or sprayed on clothing to provide protection.

CHAPTER 3

....

ACCENTUATE BEAUTY

....

80. ACNE

Acne is a skin condition that results in pimples, blackheads, white-heads, cysts, nodules, and papules. It often appears on the face but can also show up on the neck, chest, back, upper arms, shoulder, and buttocks. Acne is the most common skin problem in the United States. It happens when dead skin cells stick together with sebum (oil) inside the pore, becoming trapped. Bacteria living on the skin can sometimes get stuck in the pores with the dead skin cells. This provides a perfect breeding ground for them, and they quickly multiply. The skin becomes inflamed. If the acne goes deeper into the skin, a nodule or cyst forms. Typically, acne appears in teenagers and young adults, but it can affect anyone, even babies. Scars and dark spots on the skin can result. Mild acne can be treated with over-the-counter products that contain ben-zoyl peroxide or salicylic acid. It takes four to eight weeks of using the product for acne to clear. For best resolution, a dermatologist should treat more severe cases. Prescription-grade topical treat-ments, whole body treatments like antibiotics, or office procedures involving lasers, lights, or chemicals may be used.

Propionibacterium acnes, commonly found on the skin, is the primary bacterium responsible for acne. Antibacterial agents are needed to reduce acne, but current topical treatments often cause skin dryness and irritation. Curcumin is able to significantly inhibit the growth of *Propionibacterium acnes* bacteria on the skin and in the pores[137] and does so in a gentler way. When combined with other herbs in a facewash gel, it proved to be similar to clin-damycin gel, an antibiotic used to treat bacterial skin infections.[138]

Curcumin also reduces inflammation and can lessen the size, redness, and pain of bumps.

ACNE SPOT TREATMENT

1. Mix 1/2 teaspoon of ground turmeric with 1 teaspoon of raw honey.
2. Dab onto pimples before bed.

TURMERIC ACNE MASK

1. Mix 1 teaspoon of ground turmeric with 2 tablespoons of plain yogurt.
2. Clean the skin and apply to the affected area for 15 minutes. Wash off. Reapply a few times a week.

81. AGE SPOTS

Spending a lot of time outdoors is a healthy way to grow up, but all those years of sun exposure without sun protection can cause the appearance of brown, grey, or black, flat areas of pigmentation on the skin called age spots. They typically appear on the areas of the skin most exposed to the sun, like the face, hands, arms, chest, and shoulders. Ultraviolet radiation from the sun speeds up the production of melanin, creating darker pigmentation of the skin known as a tan. After many years of sun exposure, melanin pigments can become clumped together to form these age spots. They are generally harmless, but some people opt to treat them for cosmetic reasons. Prescription-strength creams containing retinol or hydroquinone are effective at fading the age spots.

Microdermabrasion, laser treatments, chemical peels, and light therapy are also used.

A simple at-home treatment to prevent the development of age spots is to apply turmeric. Curcumin in turmeric inhibits a specific protein and enzyme needed for the creation of melanin. The higher the dose of curcumin, the greater the inhibitory effect. It works by another method as well: by activating biochemical pathways that suppress melanin production.[139]

PREVENTATIVE HAND TREATMENT FoR AGE SPoTS

1. Mix 1/4 teaspoon of ground turmeric with 2 tablespoons of milk.
2. Rub over the back of the hands and allow mixture to remain there for 15 minutes. This will be runny, so do this treatment over the sink.
3. Rinse off. Repeat every day to prevent the formation of age spots.

82. AGING

The process of getting older involves many changes in the body. Arteries stiffen, bones lose density, memory declines, skin thins, and wrinkles appear. The rate at which these processes take place varies from person to person. Genetics and illness play a role in when and how we age, but our diet and lifestyle significantly impact the process. There are many theories of aging, but the free radical theory is growing in popularity as an explanation. It is thought that free radicals are responsible for age-related damage of cells and tissues. Free radicals are unstable molecules actively looking for an electron. They attack the nearest stable molecule and steal one of their electrons, making that molecule a free radical as well. This begins a chain reaction of creating free radicals that ultimately can destroy the cell.

The key to stopping these free radicals lies in the presence of antioxidants. Curcumin is an antioxidant that can be used to slow the aging process by preventing the activity and generation of free radicals. Because it has low bioavailability, encapsulating curcumin in elastic vesicles enables biologically active doses to be delivered to photodamaged skin. Topical application of these curcumin vesicles significantly reduced skin aging upon exposure to ultraviolet light compared to free curcumin applied in an ointment.[140] As to overall body aging, low-grade inflammation is thought to play a role. This process is driven by oxygen stress initiated by the presence of reactive oxygen species. Curcumin has a dual job here: it can remove free radicals, and it can block NF-κB, a protein complex that plays a role in the expression of proinflammatory compounds.[141] This lowers both oxygen stress and inflammation in the body and can slow down aging and decrease the probability of acquiring age-related diseases.

83. BRUISES

Often bruises happen from events that go unnoticed, such as bumping into a bedpost or catching a hip on the kitchen counter. Others happen from vigorous exercise, bleeding disorders, or blood-thinning medications. Elderly persons are more susceptible to bruises because they have thinner skin that gives less support to the blood vessels underneath. When the skin in injured, the blood

HEALTH

WELLNESS

BEAUTY

CRAFTS

cells under the skin are damaged. They leak blood, which pools underneath the surface of the skin, giving rise to a tender and sometimes painful black or blue mark. The bruise begins to heal and turns yellow or green. It eventually fades as the blood is reabsorbed. Ice and later heat can be applied to the bruise to reduce swelling and improve circulation to the area.

One of the many ways turmeric has traditionally been used in India is to treat bruises. Consuming turmeric daily can decrease inflammation in bruised areas of the body. Applying a topical paste directly to the bruise can also bring down swelling and reduce tenderness and pain. It is thought to increase circulation and can remove old blood from the injured tissue and bring nutrients to help the healing process. Curcumin has been shown to increase the production of new blood vessels and connective tissue, necessary steps to replace the damaged tissue of the bruise.[142]

BRuiSE TREATMENT

1. Mix 1 teaspoon of ground turmeric with 1 tablespoon of plain yogurt. Spread over the bruise in a thin layer.
2. After twenty minutes, rinse off. Repeat daily until the bruise has healed.

84. BuRNS

Burns can be caused by sunlight, heat, chemicals, electricity, or radiation damaging the skin and possibly underlying tissues. There are three types of burns. First-degree burns affect the outer layer of skin and cause minor inflammation, redness, and pain. Second-degree burns damage the outer layer of skin and the layer underneath. They are characterized by blisters, redness, and pain. Third-degree burns are the most serious and damage the deepest layer of skin tissue. They have a white, leathery appearance. Treatment for minor burns includes cleaning the wound, applying antibiotic cream, and taking pain medication. More severe burns should be treated by a medical professional.

Curcumin gel can rapidly heal burns with little to no scarring.[143] The speed at which healing occurs is important because infections can set in that delay wound healing. Curcumin effectively eliminates bacterial growth in burn tissue and was similar to silver sulfadiazine cream, often used to prevent and treat wound infections in burn patients.[144] Pain associated with burns can be severe, and medications to manage this can lead to dose escalations and serious side effects if used for extended periods. Curcumin can be used to control burn pain over the long term, a benefit attributed to its anti-inflammatory activity.[145] Topical application can be applied by mixing turmeric powder with coconut oil or aloe vera gel and smoothing over the skin for thirty minutes. You may want to cover the area with gauze or an old cloth. This can be repeated several times a day. Turmeric in the diet can also help reduce inflammation and pain and speed healing of the skin.

85. CRACKED HEELS

The skin on the heels of the feet can become dry and cracked. The tissue around the rim of the heels may thicken, causing calluses. Cracks can occur in the thick calluses too, especially if there is too much weight bearing down on the fat pads under the heels in the absence of shoe support. Prolonged standing and improper footwear can increase pressure on the heels, forcing them to expand sideways. If the skin is dry, this increased pressure will cause the skin to crack. Some medical or skin conditions can dry the skin, leading to this problem. Most cases of cracked heels are just irritating, but if the condition is severe, it may become painful and unsightly.

It's important to wear proper footwear to support the foot and alleviate excessive pressure on the heels. Shoes with thick soles and closed backs are recommended. The curcumin in turmeric helps alleviate dry skin by increasing the production of new blood vessels and connective tissue[146] in the heels to help in the formation of healthy skin to replace the old, cracked skin.

CRACKED HEELS TREATMENT

1. To repair the heels, begin by debriding the callused tissue to reduce its thickness. Some cracks won't heal if this extra-tough skin is not removed.
2. Then soak the feet in a warm footbath to soften the skin. After, apply a mixture of 1/4 teaspoon ground turmeric and 1 teaspoon coconut oil to the heels.
3. Leave it on for fifteen minutes, then wash the foot with warm water and mild soap. Pat dry. This can be repeated daily.

86. DANDRUFF

Dandruff is a chronic condition marked by the flaking of skin cells on the scalp. The condition is visible as white, oily-looking flakes of skin on the hair and shoulders. It is not a dangerous condition, but it can be embarrassing for some people. Dandruff is usually worse in the fall and winter, when the scalp is subjected to the drier, cooler, outdoor air and heated indoor air, which deplete moisture in the skin.

There are various causes for dandruff. Infrequent shampooing can build up layers of dead skin cells and oil. They eventually shed as dandruff. Dry skin can give rise to small, dry dandruff flakes. Yeast on the scalp can irritate the skin and lead to an overproduction of skin cells, which also flake off as dandruff. One of the most common causes of dandruff is seborrheic dermatitis. This is a condition in which oily skin is covered in flaky white or yellow scales. Mild cases are easy to treat with daily cleansing to reduce oil and skin cell buildup. Other cases are more difficult and may need medicated shampoos. Some shampoos contain antifungal and antibacterial agents to kill the microbes. Others work by slowing the death rate of skin cells to reduce buildup and flaking.

Curcumin has antifungal properties and may be used to treat dandruff from fungal pathogens. It can also increase the formation of new blood vessels and increase circulation to the scalp, bringing nutrients and stimulating the production of new skin cells to replace the old, flaky ones.

DANDRUFF TREATMENT

1. Heat 2 tablespoons of coconut oil so that it is warm to the touch. Add 1/8 teaspoon of ground turmeric and mix well.
2. Massage the oil and spice into the scalp. Wrap hair in a plastic cap or an old towel that you don't mind getting stained with turmeric.
3. Leave on for twenty minutes, then shampoo the hair as normal. Use this treatment twice a week until the dandruff clears.

HEALTH

WELLNESS

BEAUTY

CRAFTS

87. HYPERTROPHIC SCARS

A hypertrophic scar is a thickened and permanent patch of skin that forms over a wound (for instance, an injury from a cut, scrape, sore, burn, or pimple) to the deep layers of the skin. The hypertrophic scars tend to look more pronounced at the beginning but can slowly fade and improve over time. They never, however, go away. They are typically red or pink in color and slightly raised due to excess amounts of collagen produced during repair. During healing, they can be inflamed, itchy, or even painful. Some scars are small and not bothersome to the person. Others are larger or in conspicuous places like the face. These can make a person feel self-conscious or unattractive.

There are a number of procedures to reduce the appearance of scars. Chemical peels, dermabrasion, and laser therapy are a few. These require trips to the doctor and can be expensive. There is also a risk of side effects, including infection, redness, pain, and bruising.

Curcumin has a proven role in healing injured tissue. Consuming turmeric in the diet or taking curcumin supplements can help new skin cells grow, new blood vessels form, connective tissue to develop, and collagen to synthesize at the site of injury.[147] This begins the process of laying down new, healthy tissue to fill the wound and replace the old, injured tissue. Curcumin can also be used to reduce inflammation, pain, and itching.[148] Decreasing these symptoms can bring relief during the healing process. A study evaluating the effects of curcumin on hypertrophic scarring in wounded rabbit ears found that after twenty-eight days, scarring was significantly reduced.[149] Turmeric, then, can help begin the healing process, reduce unpleasant symptoms associated with healing, and diminish the look of hypertrophic scars.

88. INSECT BITES

In spring and early summer, bug bites can make sitting outside intolerable. Wearing bug repellent, long sleeves, and pants or staying inside can reduce or prevent bites, but these precautions are not foolproof. Once bitten, the skin can swell, turn red, sting, and be itchy. The insects break the skin to reach the blood that they need for nourishing and developing their eggs. Many secrete anticoagulants in their saliva to keep the blood flowing while they are trying to get a meal. The body reacts to these compounds by releasing histamines to combat the foreign substance. The blood vessels expand and irritate the nerves, causing the characteristic red, swollen, itchy bump.

Most reactions are minor and disappear in a day or two. The itching, however, can be very uncomfortable and disrupt daily living and sleep. Turmeric essential oil mixed with a carrier oil can be sprayed directly onto the skin to reduce swelling, redness, and itching.

This oil can also be used to repel insects, specifically the pesky mosquito. Turmeric oil combined with vanillin repelled three different mosquito species in both mosquito cages and large rooms for up to eight hours. This is similar to the protection of DEET—the most common insect repellent—and can be used alongside or in place of it as a topical mosquito repellent.[150]

HEALTH

WELLNESS

BEAUTY

CRAFTS

89. ITCHY SKIN

Itchy skin can be very uncomfortable and make you want to scratch. Itches can be localized to a specific area or generalized and occur all over the body. One of the most common causes is simply dry skin, and this is easily improved by adding moisture with creams, lotions, and oils. Other causes cannot be resolved so easily. These include itches from allergic reactions, medications, diseases, emotional issues, and skin conditions like eczema. Sometimes itchy skin is accompanied by bumps, rashes, blisters, or red and inflamed skin. Scratching the itch provides temporary relief but can injure the skin, causing it to look red and raw and, in some cases, become inflamed and bleed. This can lead to infection. Anti-itch creams and lotions can temporarily dull the itch, or cold compresses can quiet the nerve fibers, since the sensations of coldness and itchiness travel along the same nerves.

Many treatments do not provide patients with adequate relief from itching and produce significant side effects. A safe alternative is turmeric, even in people with compromised immune systems. One such group are hemodialysis patients. They commonly suffer from chronic itching that can severely affect their quality of life. A trial involving the administration of turmeric or placebo to hemodialysis patients noted significantly higher reductions in inflammatory proteins and an overall reduction in itching scores, as determined by the patients. No side effects from turmeric use were observed.[151] Even chronic itch from skin damage due to chemical exposure, such as mustard gas, benefits from curcumin treatment. Iranian veterans randomized to receive either curcumin or placebo for four weeks had significantly different results. No improvements were seen in the placebo group, while the curcumin group reported decreased severity of itching and an improvement in their quality of lives.[152] Generalized itching, such as from allergies, can also be helped by curcumin.[153]

90. MALE PATTERN BALDNESS

Hair grows everywhere on the body except the palms of the hands and the soles of the feet. Countless hours and money are spent trying to get rid of hair on the body, yet every hair on the head is clung to as if it were made of gold. Healthy, shiny, lustrous hair is a sign of beauty and a point of fashion and personal expression. Hair loss is common in men and can even happen in women and children. As excessive hair falls out and bald spots appear, a person may undergo significant anxiety and feel exposed, inadequate, or unattractive.

Balding happens when hair follicles on the head no longer produce new hair cells. Heredity plays a large role in hair loss and affects the age it begins, the rate at which it occurs, and the pattern it takes. Medications, disease, and hormone changes may also cause excessive hair loss. To counteract hair loss, people use medications to try to stimulate growth or slow loss. Others undergo surgery and transplant tiny plugs of skin containing hairs into the scalp. These come with side effects like rapid heart rate, sexual dysfunction, pain, infection, and scarring.

Curcumin is a potent 5-alpha-reductase inhibitor.[154] 5-alpha-reductase is an enzyme in the body that converts testosterone into the hormone dihydrotestosterone, the hormone that causes hair loss in men. By inhibiting the production of this enzyme, hair loss can be slowed or even halted.

SCALP MASK

1. Mix together 2 tablespoons of ground turmeric, 3 tablespoons of milk, and 1 teaspoon of honey.
2. Apply the paste to the scalp for thirty minutes. Wash off and repeat this two times a week.

91. OILY SKIN

The sebaceous glands beneath the skin secrete sebum through the pores to the surface of the skin. Sebum is an oily substance that protects and moisturizes the skin. When too much sebum is produced, the skin looks shiny and oily. While a healthy glow is considered attractive and youthful, a reflective sheen most definitely isn't. Too much oil can also clog pores and cause acne. Oil production varies from day to day and season to season. Hormones, mood, weather changes, stress, and genetics all play a role in sebum production. The best way to cut down on excess oil is to use a gentle cleanser on the skin every morning and night. Adding toners or acids like benzoyl peroxide or salicylic acid can help reduce oily skin, but these can be very irritating. Blotting paper and masks can draw out oil and reduce shine. If these measures aren't enough, a dermatologist can perform chemical peels or use lasers to reduce oiliness.

Oils are one of our natural anti-aging tools, so it's important not to eradicate all oils from the skin—just to reduce excessive amounts. Because many of the oil-reducing products are irritating to the skin, using natural alternatives like turmeric can be an effective and gentle method to reduce oil while preserving skin integrity. A cream formulation with turmeric extract added significantly reduced sebum production on the face after just four weeks of use, compared to the same cream without turmeric.[155]

HOMEMADE TURMERIC MASK FOR OILY SKIN

1. Mix 1/4 teaspoon ground turmeric with 1 tablespoon of gram flour and enough water to make a paste.
2. Spread over the face and allow to dry for about ten minutes. Rinse off. Some skin types will retain a slight yellow color, but this will fade. You may want to test this mask on an inconspicuous part of the body to determine if any yellow stain remains on the skin.

92. TEETH WHITENER

Bright white teeth make for a beautiful smile and give a younger and healthier appearance. There are many products in stores that claim to whiten teeth. Whitening toothpastes remove surface stains with mild abrasive agents and can achieve about one shade of difference. Some mouthwashes contain ingredients to whiten teeth, but they are less effective, and results are often not seen for twelve weeks. Whitening gels, strips, and trays contain hydrogen peroxide or other bleaching agents, which lighten deep within the tooth.

HEALTH

WELLNESS

BEAUTY

CRAFTS

Results usually last about four months. Dentists can also dramatically whiten teeth in their offices in one visit. Tooth sensitivity and tissue irritation are a few side effects of the bleaching process.

It may seem like a bad idea to put turmeric on your teeth to whiten them; after all, it seems to stain almost everything it comes into contact with. Teeth, however, are not one of these. In fact, turmeric can be used on its own or with other ingredients to whiten and brighten a smile. The final effect will differ with each person, depending on the type and depth of staining. Also bear in mind that doing this will turn the bristles of your toothbrush yellow, but you might find this to be well worth it.

TURMERIC TOOTH WHITENER

1. Mix 1 teaspoon of ground turmeric with 1/2 teaspoon of coconut oil. Put a pea-sized amount on your toothbrush and brush as normal.
2. When finished, allow the turmeric to sit on the teeth for a few minutes, then rinse thoroughly with water. Brush again with your regular toothpaste. This can be done daily.

93. UNDER-EYE CIRCLES

Dark semi-circles of skin underneath the eye can make a person look tired and haggard. There are several explanations as to why some people are unfortunate enough to have them. Because the skin underneath the eye is thin and delicate, the superficial blood vessels beneath the surface of the skin sometimes show through and give the purplish appearance of dark circles. Aging can hollow out the area below the eyes, creating shadows where volume has been depleted. Fluid can collect underneath the eye and cause swelling, which creates shadows and gives the appearance of dark circles. One common symptom of allergies is dark under-eye circles. Removing contact with the allergen can resolve the issue in these cases. Under-eye circles can also run in families. If one or both parents have under-eye discoloration, there is a greater chance that the child will too.

To minimize the appearance of dark circles, make sure to get enough sleep, stay hydrated, and wear sunscreen to prevent sun damage that can contribute to the problem. Eye creams and concealers can temporarily mask dark under-eye circles. For longer-lasting solutions, dermatologists can apply fillers or treat the area with vascular lasers. These treatments can be expensive and may not work for everyone. An inexpensive remedy that can be done at home is to use turmeric. The antioxidant and anti-inflammatory properties of turmeric both protect the skin and reduce puffiness. While nothing will totally eliminate dark circles, this treatment provides a color correction that certainly lightens the area for a brighter, fresher look.

DARK CIRCLE CORRECTOR

1. Combine 1 teaspoon of ground turmeric with 2 teaspoons of pineapple juice. Mix to form a thin paste.
2. Apply onto the dark area under the eyes, being careful to confine the paste to that area. It can be a little runny, so you may want to have a tissue ready to catch any liquid if it threatens to drip down your face.

HEALTH

WELLNESS

BEAUTY

CRAFTS

3. Wait ten to fifteen minutes, then rinse off with an old wash-cloth dipped in warm water.

94. VITILIGO

Vitiligo is a long-term condition that causes loss of the body's natural pigment and color. It occurs when melanin-producing cells die. Pigment can disappear anywhere on the body, including the skin, inside of the mouth, eyes, and hair. Most people suffer from color loss on their skin, and it can occur in a small area or over the whole body. There are two types: segmental and non-segmental. The former is less common and only appears on one segment of the body, often progressing for a short time before stopping. The latter affects both sides of the body, and color loss tends to expand over time. While most people with vitiligo do not experience any other symptoms, some have reported pain and itchiness in the affected areas. Many people apply cosmetics to the skin to camouflage the area, while others take medication or undergo light therapy or even surgery to replace lost pigment and restore the skin to its natural state of color.

One of the common therapies effective for many patients involves excimer laser treatments, a form of ultraviolet laser that can treat small areas of the skin. Combining this laser treatment with topical treatments may be more powerful than the laser alone. This was studied in ten subjects with vitiligo. They were treated with the laser treatment alone or with the laser treatment combined with tetrahydrocurcuminoid cream. Tetrahydrocurcuminoid is a compound derived from curcumin found in turmeric. After twelve weeks of treatments, both groups saw significant repigmentation, although the group receiving the tetrahydrocurcuminoid cream had slightly better results.[156] Any improvement, even slight ones, can have a powerful impact on the patient's confidence and overall well-being.

HEALTH

WELLNESS

BEAUTY

CRAFTS

CHAPTER 4

APPLY IN ARTS AND CRAFTS

HEALTH

WELLNESS

BEAUTY

CRAFTS

95. EASTER EGGS

The practice of decorating eggshells goes back thousands of years. Ostrich eggs were decorated in gold and silver and placed in graves as symbols of death and rebirth. Our modern tradition of dying chicken eggshells began with the Christians of Mesopotamia, who stained eggs red in memory of the blood of Christ. The Christian church adopted the practice and used the eggs as a symbol of the resurrection of Jesus. This Easter-time custom spread throughout Christendom. Today, chicken eggs are stained many colors, some with intricate decorations and beautiful designs. Easter eggs today also include foil-wrapped chocolate eggs and hollow plastic eggs filled with candy.

Dyeing chicken eggs during the Easter season has become a widespread practice in many households and provides a fun, albeit messy, activity for children and adults alike. Eggs are hardboiled then cooled. Different color dyes are prepared in various dishes, and the eggs are placed into the dye for several minutes to hours. The shell absorbs the dye and becomes stained with the color. Artificial coloring is often added to water to achieve this look, but natural dyes can also be used. Turmeric imparts a beautiful golden-yellow color to eggshells.

TURMERIC EASTER EGG DYE

1. Heat 2 cups of water over medium-high heat, then add 2 teaspoons of vinegar and 1 teaspoon of salt.
2. When the salt dissolves, add in 3 tablespoons of ground turmeric and mix.

3. Simmer for a few minutes, then remove from the stove. Pour the golden liquid into a glass container and add the room-temperature hardboiled eggs. The longer the eggs soak in the liquid, the more vibrant the color will be.

96. MIMOSAS

A popular cocktail served at brunches or weddings is the mimosa. It is traditionally served in a champagne flute with equal parts champagne or sparkling wine and orange juice. Variations of this drink commonly increase the champagne-to-juice ratio or substitute other juices like pineapple or cranberry for orange. To spice up this drink and add a healthful boost, add a pinch of turmeric powder or a small amount of fresh, grated turmeric root. Not only will the color of the drink intensify and thus appeal to the eyes, your body will love turmeric's antioxidant, anti-inflammatory, antimicrobial, and wound-healing properties.

97. NON-TOXIC FOOD DYE

Artificial colors have long been added to food to make them more visually appealing. After all, salmon doesn't always look so pink, pickles so green, or cheese so orange. It's not just added to natural foods, either. Food coloring is added to cereal, pasta, Jell-O, juice, chips, and cakes. The list is seemingly endless. Currently, seven FDA dyes are approved for use in food in the United States: FD&C Blue No. 1, FD&C Blue No. 2, FD&C Green No. 3, FD&C

HEALTH

WELLNESS

BEAUTY

CRAFTS

Red No. 3, FD&C Red No. 40, FD&C Yellow No. 5, and FD&C Yellow No. 6. This list has dwindled down from eighty since the early twentieth century due to adverse health concerns. Even the list of seven is under scrutiny, but conflicting scientific studies are preventing the FDA from further bans.

The public is increasingly looking to avoid artificial dyes, and many companies are now searching for natural alternatives that are safe and non-toxic. Turmeric can be used as a yellow food dye for rice, frosting, cakes, sauces, mustards, relishes, and anything else you want to be yellow. It takes a greater amount than artificial dyes, but still, the little amount used won't impart any flavor in the food, just the color. Begin by adding a small amount of turmeric dye and increase to reach the desired shade of yellow.

YELLOW FOOD DYE FOR SAVORY DISHES

1. Boil 1/2 cup of water and add 1 teaspoon of ground turmeric. Mix and allow it to simmer for five minutes. Take off the stove and cool.
2. Use as desired, remembering to account for the extra volume being added with the dye. The remaining coloring can be stored in the refrigerator for up to two weeks.

CONCENTRATED YELLOW FOOD DYE FOR SWEET TREATS

1. Boil 1 cup of water and add 5 tablespoons of sugar and 2 teaspoons of ground turmeric.
2. When the sugar has dissolved, simmer over low heat until half the liquid has evaporated. Cool and use.

98. POPSICLES

Popsicles, also known as ice pops or freezer pops, are a favorite summertime treat to quench the thirst and cool the body. They are made by freezing fruit juices or other water-based flavored liquids around a stick. Many of the commercial brands use artificial colors and flavors to make the brightly colored treats. All-natural versions are easy to make at home using a base of yogurt, juice, flavored water, or any freezable beverage. Adding combinations of fruit, vegetables, spices, nuts, or herbs can produce wonderful concoctions. Molds in various shapes and sizes can be purchased and used at home, but ice cube trays and small freezable cups can also be used. The beauty of molds is that they come with sticks and trays for an easy and tidy setup. The popsicles also tend to slide out of the molds fairly effortlessly.

Popsicles aren't just for children. Turmeric popsicles are a delicious frozen treat for adults and children alike and provide an enjoyable and convenient way to consume turmeric in the diet and reap all the healthful benefits.

TURMERIC MANGO POPSICLES

1 cup unsweetened coconut milk
1/2 cup fresh chopped mango
2 tablespoons honey
1 teaspoon ground turmeric
1/2 teaspoon ground ginger
1/2 teaspoon vanilla
dash of black pepper

1. Mix in a blender until smooth.
2. Pour into popsicle molds and freeze for several hours until ready.

99. TEMPoRARY TATTOOS

The practice of tattooing is an ancient one that spans many centuries and cultures. Today, tattoos have become increasingly popular, with 20 percent of Americans having at least one. Dye is injected by a mechanized needle into the dermis below the top layer of skin. Because the skin is injured, the body reacts by causing swelling, redness, and pain in the area in an attempt to remove what the body perceives as foreign particles. Much of the pigment is left behind during the healing process, however, leaving a permanent tattoo. For those that want the beauty and decorative value that a tattoo brings without committing to a lifelong design, temporary tattoos are the answer. These use natural dyes painted onto the surface of the skin that leave a stain lasting for several days to several weeks.

One of the most popular methods of applying temporary tattoos is to use henna, a plant whose dried and powdered leaves can be made into a paste. The paste is painted onto the hands and feet (and other body parts, if desired) in intricate designs. The longer it is left on, the darker the stain will be. At first, the color will be orange, but in a few days, the henna tattoo will darken to a deep reddish brown. Turmeric can then be used to enhance the beauty of the tattoo by adding a beautiful yellow color to areas of the design.

This requires a paintbrush to be dampened in water and mixed directly with turmeric powder. Parts of the tattoo can be carefully filled in with the turmeric. Allow it to dry, then rub off any excess powder. Apply another coat with the paintbrush. Do this several times until the desired shade is reached. This color should last about two days. Turmeric can also be used as the primary or only dye to create patterns. Mix with water and apply to the skin with a thin-tipped brush or a small applicator bottle with a plastic or metal tip.

100. TIE-DYED T-SHIRT

Tie-dye is a term used to describe the process of partially or wholly coloring fabric with various colors and designs. The fabric is folded, twisted, or crumpled and tied at strategic places using rubber bands or string. Dye is then added to some or all of the garment, usually in bright, bold colors. Even though the earliest examples of tie-dyed clothing originated 1,500 years ago, it wasn't until the late 1960s that tie-dying became a fad born of the psychedelic music era, and it never really went away. Tie-dyed T-shirts, pant, skirts, scarves, and hats can be found in all manner of shops. There are many home kits that anyone can purchase to decorate their own clothing, but a very inexpensive way to do so is by harnessing the natural dye of turmeric—that is, if you want a yellow tie-dyed creation. Natural fibers work best, so choose clothing that is 100% cotton, hemp, linen, wool, or silk. By far, cotton is the most commonly used fabric.

TIE-DYED T-SHIRT

1. Wash a new or old white 100 percent cotton T-shirt. Do not use fabric softener because it will coat the fibers and prevent them from fully absorbing the dye.

2. Fill a large stainless steel pot with water and vinegar in a 4:1 ratio. Place the T-shirt into the pot over medium-low heat for an hour. This will assist the fibers in holding the dye through many washes.

3. After an hour, remove the T-shirt and rinse over the sink until the vinegar smell has disappeared.

4. When dry, lay the T-shirt flat. Beginning at the middle, wrap an elastic band around about two inches of fabric. Gather two more inches of fabric below the first elastic and add another one. Do this until the entire T-shirt is wrapped in elastics, equally spaced about two inches apart.

5. Rinse and fill the pot with water again. This time, add ground turmeric and mix thoroughly. The more you add, the brighter yellow your T-shirt will be. Begin with a few tablespoons and add more for a stronger color, if desired. Bring to a low simmer on the stove for twenty minutes.

6. Reduce heat to low and add the T-shirt. Allow the T-shirt to absorb the yellow dye for between thirty minutes to an hour, stirring occasionally.

7. Remove the pot from the heat and let it cool for fifteen minutes.

8. Take the T-shirt out, and rinse it in cold water until it runs clear. Remove the rubber bands and rinse again. The T-shirt is now ready to be dried and worn.

9. Wash the T-shirt on its own the first few times, as small amount of dye may come out of the garment.

101. YELLOW PLAYDOUGH

Play-Doh, the children's toy that was eventually named in the "Century of Toys List" by the Toy Industry Association in 2003, was first developed as a wallpaper cleaner in the 1930s. With the advent of washable vinyl wallpaper and the switch from coal-based heating to natural gas, its use as a cleaner became obsolete. The product was re-marketed as a child's modeling toy that was safe and non-toxic, didn't stain fingers or clothes, and was reusable. Now that's a toy parents can get behind! Since then, other brands have emerged onto the market, and they can be found in an array of bright colors.

Playdough is primarily made of water, flour, and salt. The commercial brand, Play-Doh, also contains binders, preservatives, artificial fragrances, and colors, among other ingredients. Since it is usually children playing with this toy and because of their penchant for eating it, making playdough at home with all-natural ingredients from the kitchen can give parents peace of mind, knowing their children aren't consuming anything that could potentially be harmful. Beet juice can be used for red coloring, paprika for orange, spirulina powder for green, blackberries for purple, and turmeric for yellow.

YELLOW PLAYDOUGH RECIPE

1/2 cup water
1/2 teaspoon ground turmeric or 1/2 tablespoon grated fresh turmeric
1/2 cup flour
1/4 cup salt

1/2 tablespoon cream of tartar
1/2 tablespoon olive oil

1. *Turmeric water:* Pour 1/2 cup of water into a pot on the stove and add 1/2 teaspoon of ground turmeric or 1/2 tablespoon grated fresh turmeric. Bring to a boil and simmer for ten minutes. Strain through a fine sieve.

2. *Playdough:* Combine the flour, salt, and cream of tartar in a bowl. Add the olive oil to the turmeric water, then mix in the dry ingredients. Stir constantly until a soft dough forms and pulls away from the sides of the pot (approximately three to five minutes). Allow the dough to cool enough to be comfortably handled. Transfer the dough to a floured surface, and knead until a firm ball forms. Store in an airtight container.

HEALTH

WELLNESS

BEAUTY

CRAFTS

NOTES

1. Polasa, K., B. Sesikaran, T. P. Krishna, and K. Krishnaswamy. 1991. "Turmeric (*Curcuma longa*)-induced reduction in urinary mutagens." *Food and Chemical Toxicology* 29: 699–706.

2. Oppenheimer, A. 1937. "Turmeric (curcumin) in biliary diseases." *Lancet* 229: 619–621.

3. Esatbeyoglu, T., K. Ulbrich, C. Rehberg, S. Rohn, and G. Rimbach. 2015. "Thermal stability, antioxidant, and anti-inflammatory activity of curcumin and its degradation product 4-vinyl guaiacol." *Food & Function* 6 (3): 887–893.

4. Borde, Vinod Uttamrao. 2011. "Effect of boiling and roasting on the antioxidants concentrations in extracts of fresh ginger (*Zingiber officinale*) and turmeric (*Curcuma longa*)." *International Journal of Ayurvedic and Herbal Medicine* 1: 2.

5. Shoba, G., D. Joy, T. Joseph, M. Majeed, R. Rajendran, and P. S. Srinivas. 1998. "Influence of piperine on the pharmacokinetics of curcumin in animals and human volunteers." *Planta Medica* 64 (4): 353–356.

6. Lao, C. D., M. T. Ruffin, D. Normolle, D. D. Heath, S. I. Murray, J. M. Bailey, M. E. Boggs, J. Crowell, C. L. Rock, and D. E. Brenner. 2006. "Dose escalation of a curcuminoid formulation." *BMC Complementary and Alternative Medicine* 17 (6): 10.

7. Barthelemy, S., L. Vergnes, M. Moynier, D. Guyot, S. Labidalle, and E. Bahraoui. 1998. "Curcumin and curcumin derivatives inhibit Tat-mediated trans-activation of type 1 human immunodeficiency virus long terminal repeat." *Research in Virology* 149 (1): 43–52.

8. Vajragupta, O., P. Boonchoong, G. M. Morris, and A. J. Olson. 2005. "Active site binding modes of curcumin in HIV-1 protease and integrase." *Bioorganic & Medicinal Chemistry Letters* 15 (14): 3364–3368.

9. Mazumder, A., K. Raghavan, J. Weinstein, K. W. Kohn, and Y. Pommier. 1995. "Inhibition of human immunodeficiency virus type-1 integrase by curcumin." *Biochemical Pharmacology* 49 (8): 1165–1170.

10. Balasubramanyam, K., R. A. Varier, M. Altaf, V. Swaminathan, N. B. Siddappa, U. Ranga, and T. K. Kundu. 2004. "Curcumin, a novel p300/CREB-binding protein-specific inhibitor of acetyltransferase, represses the acetylation of

histone/nonhistone proteins and histone acetyltransferase-dependent chromatin transcription." *Journal of Biological Chemistry* 279 (49): 51163–51171.

11. Shin, H. S., H. J. See, S. Y. Jung, D. W. Choi, D. A. Kwon, M. J. Bae, K. S. Sung, and D. H. Shon. 2015. "Turmeric (*Curcuma longa*) attenuates food allergy symptoms by regulating type 1/type 2 helper T cells (Th1/Th1) balance in a mouse model of food allergy." *Journal of Ethnopharmacology* 175: 21–29.

12. Kobayashi, T., S. Hashimoto, and T. Horie. 1997. "Curcumin inhibition of Dermatophagoides farinea-induced interleukin-5 (IL-5) and granulocyte macrophage-colony stimulating factor (GM-CSF) production by lymphocytes from bronchial asthmatics." *Biochemical Pharmacology* 54 (7): 819–824.

13. Wu, S., and D. Xiao. 2016. "Effect of curcumin on nasal symptoms and airflow in patients with perennial allergic rhinitis." *Annals of Allergy, Asthma and Immunology* 117 (6): 697–702.

14. Baum, L., C. W. Lam, S. K. Cheung, T. Kwok, V. Lui, J. Tsoh, L. Lam, V. Leung, E. Hui, C. Ng, J. Woo, H. F. Chiu, W. B. Goggins, B. C. Zee, K. F. Cheng, C. Y. Fong, A. Wong, H. Mok, M. S. Chow, P. C. Ho, S. P. Ip, C. S. Ho, X. W. Yu, C. Y. Lai, M. H. Chan, S. Szeto, I. H. Chan, and V. Mok. 2008. "Six-month randomized, placebo-controlled, double-blind, pilot clinical trial of curcumin in patients with Alzheimer disease." *Journal of Clinical Psychopharmacology* 28 (1): 110–113.

15. Ram, A., M. Das, and B. Ghosh. 2003. "Curcumin attenuates allergen-induced airway hyperresponsiveness in sensitized guinea pigs." *Biological and Pharmaceutical Bulletin* 26 (7): 1021–4.

16. Ramírez-Tortosa, M. C., M. D. Mesa, M. C. Aguilera, J. L. Quiles, L. Baró, C. L. Ramirez-Tortosa, E. Martinez-Victoria, and A. Gil. 1999. "Oral administration of a turmeric extract inhibits LDL oxidation and has hypocholesterolemic effects in rabbits with experimental atherosclerosis." *Atherosclerosis* 147 (2): 371–378.

17. Olszanecki, R., J. Jawień, M. Gajda, L. Mateuszuk, A. Gebska, M. Korabiowska, S. Chłopicki, and R. Korbut. 2005. "Effect of curcumin on atherosclerosis in apoE/LDLR-double knockout mice." *Journal of Physiology and Pharmacology* 56 (4): 627–35.

18. Ghaffari, S. B., M. H. Sarrafzadeh, Z. Fakhroueian, S. Shahriari, and M. R. Khorramizadeh. 2017. "Functionalization of ZnO nanoparticles by 3-mercaptopropionic acid for aqueous curcumin delivery: Synthesis, characterization, and anticancer assessment." *Materials Science and Engineering C: Materials for Biological Applications* 79: 465–472.

19. Obata, K., T. Kojima, T. Masaki, T. Okabayashi, S. Yokota, S. Hirakawa, K. Nomura, A. Takasawa, M. Murata, S. Tanaka, J. Fuchimoto, N. Fujii, H.

Tsutsumi, T. Himi, and N. Sawada. 2013. "Curcumin prevents replication of respiratory syncytial virus and the epithelial responses to it in human nasal epithelial cells." *PLoS One* 8 (9): e70225.

20. Neelofar, K., S. Shreaz, B. Rimple, S. Muralidhar, M. Nikhat, and L. A. Khan. 2011. "Curcumin as a promising anticandidal of clinical interest." *Canadian Journal of Microbiology* 57 (3): 204–210.

21. Farhangkhoee, H., Z. A. Khan, S. Chen, and S. Chakrabarti. 2006. "Differential effects of curcumin on vasoactive factors in the diabetic rat heart." *Nutrition and Metabolism* (London) 3: 27.

22. Feng, B., S. Chen, J. Chiu, B. George, and S. Chakrabarti. 2008. "Regulation of cardiomyocyte hypertrophy in diabetes at the transcriptional level." *American Journal of Physiology-Endocrinology and Metabolism* 294 (6): E1119–1126.

23. Suryanarayana, P., M. Saraswat, T. Mrudula, T. P. Krishna, K. Krishnaswamy, and G. B. Reddy. 2005. "Curcumin and turmeric delay streptozotocin-induced diabetic cataract in rats." *Investigative Ophthalmology and Visual Science* 46 (6): 2092–2099.

24. Oppenheimer, "Turmeric (curcumin) in biliary diseases."

25. Marwick, J. A., K. Ito, I. M. Adcock, and P. A. Kirkham. 2007. "Oxidative stress and steroid resistance in asthma and COPD: pharmacological manipulation of HDAC-2 as a therapeutic strategy." *Expert Opinion on Therapeutic Targets* 11 (6): 745–755.

26. Cruz-Correa, M., D. A. Shoskes, P. Sanchez, R. Zhao, L. M. Hylind, S. D. Wexner, and F. M. Giardiello. 2006. "Combination treatment with curcumin and quercetin of adenomas in familial adenomatous polyposis." *Clinical Gastroenterology and Hepatology* 4 (8): 1035–1038.

27. Holt, P. R., S. Katz, and R. Kirshoff. 2005. "Curcumin therapy in inflammatory bowel disease: a pilot study." *Digestive Diseases and Sciences* 50 (11): 2191–2193.

28. Usharani, P., A. A. Mateen, M. U. Naidu, Y. S. Raju, and N. Chandra. 2008. "Effect of NCB-02, atorvastatin and placebo on endothelial function, oxidative stress and inflammatory markers in patients with type 2 diabetes mellitus: a randomized, parallel-group, placebo-controlled, 8-week study." *Drugs in R&D* 9 (4): 243–250.

29. Wickenberg, J., S. L. Ingemansson, and J. Hlebowicz. 2010. "Effects of *Curcuma longa* (turmeric) on postprandial plasma glucose and insulin in healthy subjects." *Nutrition Journal* 9: 43.

30. Chuengsamarn, S., S. Rattanamongkolgul, R. Luechapudiporn, C. Phisalaphong, and S. Jirawatnotai. 2012. "Curcumin extract for prevention of type 2 diabetes." *Diabetes Care* 35 (11): 2121–2127.

31. Srinivasan, M. 1972. "Effect of curcumin on blood sugar as seen in a diabetic subject." *Indian Journal of Medical Science* 26 (4): 269–270.

32. Nishiyama, T., T. Mae, H. Kishida, M. Tsukagawa, Y. Mimaki, M. Kuroda, Y. Sashida, K. Takahashi, T. Kawada, K. Nakagawa, and M. Kitahara. 2005. "Curcuminoids and sesquiterpenoids in turmeric (*Curcuma longa L.*) suppress an increase in blood glucose level in type 2 diabetic KK-Ay mice." *Journal of Agriculture and Food Chemistry* 53 (4): 959–963.

33. Kuhad, A., and K. Chopra. 2007. "Curcumin attenuates diabetic encephalopathy in rats: behavioral and biochemical evidences." *European Journal of Pharmacology* 576 (1–3): 34–42.

34. Usharani, P., et al., "Effect of NCB-02, atorvastatin and placebo on endothelial function, oxidative stress and inflammatory markers in patients with type 2 diabetes mellitus."

35. Smith, S. E., C. M. Man, P. K. Yip, E. Tang, A. G. Chapman, and B. S. Meldrum. 1996. "Anticonvulsant effects of 7-nitroindazole in rodents with reflex epilepsy may result from L-arginine accumulation of a reduction in nitric oxide of L-citrulline formation." *British Journal of Pharmacology* 119: 165–173.

36. Sumanont, Y., Y. Murakami, M. Tohda, O. Vajragupta, H. Watanabe, and K. Matsumoto. 2006. "Prevention of kainic acid-induced changes in nitric oxide level and neuronal cell damage in the rat hippocampus by manganese complexes of curcumin and diacetylcurcumin." *Life Science* 78 (16): 1884–1891.

37. Yun, D. G., and D. G. Lee. 2016. "Antibacterial activity of curcumin via apoptosis-like response in *Escherichia coli*." *Applied Microbiology and Biotechnology* 100 (12): 5505–5514.

38. Tyagi, P., M. Singh, H. Kumari, A. Kumari, and K. Mukhopadhyay. 2015. "Bactericidal activity of curcumin I is associated with damaging of bacterial membrane." *PLoS One* 10 (3): e0121313.

39. Centers for Disease Control and Prevention. "Genital Herpes—CDC Fact Sheet." Accessed September 13, 2017. https://www.cdc.gov/std/herpes /herpes-feb-2017.pdf.

40. Bourne, K. Z., N. Bourne, S. F. Reising, and L. R. Stanberry. 1999. "Plant products as topical microbicide candidates: assessment of *in vitro* and *in vivo* activity against herpes simplex virus type 2." *Antiviral Research* 42 (3): 219–226.

41. Waghmare, P. F., A. U. Chaudhari, V. M. Karhadkar, and A. S. Jamkhande. 2011. "Comparative evaluation of turmeric and chlorhexidine gluconate mouthwash in prevention of plaque formation and gingivitis: a clinical and microbiological study." *Journal of Contemporary Dental Practice* 12 (4): 221–224.

42. *PDR for Herbal Medicines*, 2nd edition. 2000. Montvale, New Jersey: Medical Economics Company. Page 776.

43. Kim, H. J., H. S. Yoo, J. C. Kim, C. S. Park, M. S. Choi, M. Kim, H. Choi, J. S. Min, Y. S. Kim, S. W. Yoon, and J. K. Ahn. 2009. "Antiviral effect of *Curcuma longa* Linn extract against hepatitis B virus replication." *Journal of Ethnopharmacology* 124 (2): 189–196.

44. Kim, K., K. H. Kim, H. Y. Kim, H. K. Cho, N. Sakamoto, and J. Cheong. 2010. "Curcumin inhibits hepatitis C virus replication via suppressing the Akt-SREBP-1 pathway." *FEBS Letters* 584 (4): 707–712.

45. Pashine, L., J. V. Singh, A. K. Vaish, S. K. Ojha, and A. A. Mahdi. 2012. "Effect of turmeric (*Curcuma longa*) on overweight hyperlipidemic subjects: Double blind study." *Indian Journal of Community Health* 24 (2): 113–117.

46. Alwi, I., T. Santoso, S. Suyono, B. Sutrisna, F. D. Suyatna, S. B. Kresno, and S. Ernie. 2008. "The effect of curcumin on lipid level in patients with acute coronary syndrome." *Acta Medica Indonesia* 40 (4): 201–210.

47. Centers for Disease Control and Prevention. "Genital HPV Infection—CDC Fact Sheet." Accessed September 14, 2017. https://www.cdc.gov/std/hpv/HPV-FS-July-2017.pdf.

48. Basu, P., S. Dutta, R. Begum, S. Mittal, P. D. Dutta, A. C. Bharti, C. K. Panda, J. Biswas, B. Dey, G. P. Talwar, and B. C. Das. 2013. "Clearance of cervical human papillomavirus infection by topical application of curcumin and curcumin containing polyherbal cream: a phase II randomized controlled study." *Asian Pacific Journal of Cancer Prevention* 14 (10): 5753–5759.

49. Divya, C. S., and M. R. Pillai. 2006. "Antitumor action of curcumin in human papillomavirus associated cells involves downregulation of viral oncogenes, prevention of NFkB and AP-1 translocation, and modulation of apoptosis." *Molecular Carcinogenesis* 45 (5): 320–332.

50. Chongtham, A., and N. Agrawal. 2016. "Curcumin modulates cell death and is protective in Huntington's disease model." *Scientific Reports* 6: 18736.

51. Sandhir, R., A. Yadav, A. Mehrotra, A. Sunkaria, A. Singh, and S. Sharma. 2014. "Curcumin nanoparticles attenuate neurochemical and neurobehavioral deficits in experimental model of Huntington's disease." *Neuromolecular Medicine* 16 (1): 106–118.

52. Singh, S., S. Jamwal, and P. Kumar. 2015. "Piperine enhances the protective effect of curcumin against 3-NP induced neurotoxicity: Possible neurotransmitters modulation mechanism." *Neurochemical Research* 40 (8): 1758–1766.

53. Khajehdehi, P., M. Pakfetrat, K. Javidnia, F. Azad, L. Malekmakan, M. H. Nasab, and G. Dehghanzadeh. 2011. "Oral supplementation of turmeric attenuates proteinuria, transforming growth factor-beta and interleukin-8

levels in patients with overt type 2 diabetic nephropathy: a randomized, double-blind and placebo-controlled study." *Scandinavian Journal of Urology and Nephrology* 45 (5): 365–370.

54. Zhou, X., B. Zhang, Y. Cui, S. Chen, Z. Teng, G. Lu, J. Wang, and X. Deng. 2017. "Curcumin promotes the clearance of *Listeria monocytogenes* both *in vitro* and *in vivo* by reducing listeriolysin O oligomers. *Frontiers in Immunology* 8: 574.

55. Liu, Y., Y. M. Wu, and P. Y. Zhang. 2015. "Protective effects of curcumin and quercetin during benzo(a)pyrene induced lung carcinogenesis in mice." *European Review for Medical and Pharmacological Sciences* 19: 1736–1743.

56. Khajehdehi, P., B. Zanjaninejad, E. Aflaki, M. Nazarinia, F. Azad, L. Malekmakan L, and G. R. Dehghanzadeh. 2012. "Oral supplementation of turmeric decreases proteinuria, hematuria, and systolic blood pressure in patients suffering from relapsing or refractory lupus nephritis: a randomized and placebo-controlled study." *Journal of Renal Nutrition* 22 (1): 50–57.

57. Mishra, K., A. P. Dash, B. K. Swain, and N. Dey. 2009. "Anti-malarial activities of *Andrographis paniculata* and *Hedyotis corymbosa* extracts and their combination with curcumin." *Malaria Journal* 8: 26.

58. Appendino, G., G. Belcaro, U. Cornelli, R. Luzzi, S. Togni, M. Dugall, M. R. Cesarone, B. Feragalli, E. Ippolito, B. M. Errichi, L. Pellegrini, A. Ledda, A. Ricci, P. Bavera, M. Hosoi, S. Stuard, M. Corsi, S. Errichi, and G. Gizzi. 2011. "Potential role of curcumin phytosome (Meriva) in controlling the evolution of diabetic microangiopathy. A pilot study." *Panminerva Medica* 53 (3 Suppl 1): 43–49.

59. Akyuz, S., F. Turan, L. Gurbuzler, A. Arici, E. Sogut, and O. Ozkan. 2016. "The anti-inflammatory and antioxidant effects of curcumin in middle ear infection." *Journal of Craniofacial Surgery* 27 (5): e494–497.

60. Natarajan, C., and J. J. Bright. 2002. "Curcumin inhibits experimental allergic encephalomyelitis by blocking IL-12 signaling through Janus kinase-STAT pathway in T lymphocytes." *Journal of Immunology* 168 (12): 6506–6513.

61. Chin, K. Y. 2016. "The spice for joint inflammation: anti-inflammatory role of curcumin in treating osteoarthritis." *Journal of Craniofacial Surgery* 10: 3029–3042.

62. Belcaro, G., M. R. Cesarone, M. Dugall, L. Pellegrini, A. Ledda, M. G. Grossi, S. Togni, and G. Appendino. 2010. "Product-evaluation registry of Meriva, a curcumin-phosphatidylcholine complex, for the complementary management of osteoarthritis." *Panminerva Medica* 52 (2 Suppl 1): 55–62.

63. Belcaro, G., M. R. Cesarone, M. Dugall, L. Pellegrini, A. Ledda, M. G. Grossi MG, S. Togni, and G. Appendino. 2010. "Efficacy and safety of Meriva, a

curcumin-phosphatidylcholine complex, during extended administration in osteoarthritis patients." *Alternative Medicine Review* 15 (4): 337–344.

64. Lev-Ari, S., L. Strier, D. Kazanov, O. Elkayam, D. Lichtenberg, D. Caspi, and N. Arber. 2006. "Curcumin synergistically potentiates the growth-inhibitory and pro-apoptotic effects of celecoxib in osteoarthritis synovial adherent cells." *Rheumatology* (Oxford) 45 (2): 171–177.

65. Kuptniratsaikul, V., P. Dajpratham, W. Taechaarpornkul, M. Buntragulpoontawee, P. Lukkanapichonchut, C. Chootip, J. Saengsuwan, K. Tantayakom, and S. Laongpech. 2014. "Efficacy and safety of *Curcuma domestica* extracts compared with ibuprofen in patients with knee osteoarthritis: a multicenter study." *Clinical Interventions in Aging* 9: 451–458.

66. Zbarsky, V., K. P. Datla, S. Parkar, D. K. Rai, O. I. Aruoma, and D. T. Dexter. 2005. "Neuroprotective properties of the natural phenolic antioxidants curcumin and naringenin but not quercetin and fisetin in a 6-OHDA model of Parkinson's disease." *Free Radical Research* 39 (10): 1119–1125.

67. Prucksunand, C., B. Indrasukhsri, M. Leethochawalit, and K. Hungspreugs. 2001. "Phase II clinical trial on effect of the long turmeric (*Curcuma longa linn*) on healing of peptic ulcer." *Southeast Asian Journal of Tropical Medicine and Public Health* 32 (1): 208–215.

68. Kositchaiwat, C., S. Kositchaiwat, and J. Havanondha. 1993. "*Curcuma longa linn* in the treatment of gastric ulcer comparison to liquid antacid: a controlled clinical trial." *Journal of the Medical Association of Thailand* 76 (11): 601–605.

69. Izui, S., S. Sekine, K. Maeda, M. Kuboniwa, A. Takada, A. Amano, and H. Nagata. 2016. "Antibacterial activity of curcumin against periodontopathic bacteria." *Journal of Periodontology* 87 (1): 83–90.

70. Cao, H., H. Yu, Y. Feng, L. Chen, and F. Liang. 2017. "Curcumin inhibits prostate cancer by targeting PGK1 in the FOXD3/miR-143 axis." *Cancer Chemotherapy Pharmacology* 79 (5): 985–994.

71. Thomas, R., M. Williams, H. Sharma, A. Chaudry, and P. Bellamy. 2014. "A double-blind, placebo-controlled randomised trial evaluating the effect of a polyphenol-rich whole food supplement on PSA progression in men with prostate cancer—the U.K. NCRN Pomi-T study." *Prostate Cancer and Prostatic Disease* 17 (2): 180–186.

72. Kowluru, R. A., and M. Kanwar. 2007. "Effects of curcumin on retinal oxidative stress and inflammation in diabetes." *Nutrition and Metabolism* (London) 4: 8.

73. Deodhar, S. D., R. Sethi, and R. C. Srimal. 1980. "Preliminary study on anti-rheumatic activity of curcumin (diferuloyl methane)." *Indian Journal of Medical Research* 71: 632–634.

74. Chandran, B., and A. Goel. 2012. "A randomized, pilot study to assess the efficacy and safety of curcumin in patients with active rheumatoid arthritis." *Phytotherapy Research* 26 (11): 1719–1725.

75. Funk, J. L., J. N. Oyarzo, J. B. Frye, G. Chen, R. C. Lantz, S. D. Jolad, A. M. Sólyom, and B. N. Timmermann. 2006. "Turmeric extracts containing curcuminoids prevent experimental rheumatoid arthritis." *Journal of Natural Products* 69 (3): 351–355.

76. Narayanan, A., K. Kehn-Hall, S. Senina, L. Lundberg, R. Van Duyne, I. Guendel, R. Das, A. Baer, L. Bethel, M. Turell, A. L. Hartman, B. Das, C. Bailey, and F. Kashanchi. 2012. "Curcumin inhibits Rift Valley fever virus replication in human cells." *Journal of Biological Chemistry* 287 (40): 33198–33214.

77. Bishnoi, M., K. Chopra, and S. K. Kulkarni. 2008. "Protective effect of curcumin, the active principle of turmeric (*Curcuma longa*) in haloperidol-induced orofacial dyskinesia and associated behavioural, biochemical and neurochemical changes in rat brain." *Pharmacological Biochemistry and Behavior* 88 (4): 511–522.

78. Tourkina, E., P. Gooz, J. C. Oates, A. Ludwicka-Bradley, R. M. Silver, and S. Hoffman. 2004. "Curcumin-induced apoptosis in scleroderma lung fibro-blasts: role of protein kinase [C] epsilon." *American Journal of Respiratory Cell and Molecular Biology* 31 (1): 28–35.

79. Lelli, D., C. Pedone, and A. Sahebkar. 2017. "Curcumin and treatment of melanoma: The potential role of microRNAs." *Biomedical Pharmacotherapy* 88: 832–834.

80. Jose, A., S. Labala, K. M. Ninave, S. K. Gade, and V. V. K. Venuganti. 2017. "Effective skin cancer treatment by topical co-delivery of curcumin and STAT3 siRNA using cationic liposomes." *AAPS PharmSciTech* 19 (1): 166–175.

81. Wang, J., X. Zhou, W. Li, X. Deng, Y. Deng, and X. Niu. 2016. "Curcumin protects mice from *Staphylococcus aureus* pneumonia by interfering with the self-assembly process of α-hemolysin." *Scientific Reports* 6: 28254.

82. Tyagi, P., et al., "Bactericidal activity of curcumin I is associated with damaging of bacterial membrane."

83. Teow, S. Y., and S. A. Ali. 2017. "Altered antibacterial activity of curcumin in the presence of serum albumin, plasma and whole blood." *Pakistan Journal of Pharmaceutical Science* 30 (2): 449–457.

84. Holt, P. R., S. Katz, and R. Kirshoff. 2005. "Curcumin therapy in inflammatory bowel disease: a pilot study." *Digestive Diseases and Sciences* 50 (11): 2191–2193.

85. Hanai, H., T. Iida, K. Takeuchi, F. Watanabe, Y. Maruyama, A. Andoh, T. Tsujikawa, Y. Fujiyama, K. Mitsuyama, M. Sata, M. Yamada, Y. Iwaoka, K. Kanke, H. Hiraishi, K. Hirayama, H. Arai, S. Yoshii, M. Uchijima, T. Nagata, and Y. Koide. 2006. "Curcumin maintenance therapy for ulcerative colitis: randomized, multicenter, double-blind, placebo-controlled trial." *Clinical Gastroenterology and Hepatology* 4 (12): 1502–1506.

86. Sasaki, H., Y. Sunagawa, K. Takahashi, A. Imaizumi, H. Fukuda, T. Hashimoto, H. Wada, Y. Katanasaka, H. Kakeya, M. Fujita, K. Hasegawa, and T. Morimoto. 2011. "Innovative preparation of curcumin for improved oral bioavailability." *Biological and Pharmaceutical Bulletin* 34 (5): 660–665.

87. Lopresti, A. L., and P. D. Drummond. 2017. "Efficacy of curcumin, and a saffron/curcumin combination for the treatment of major depression: A randomised, double-blind, placebo-controlled study." *Journal of Affective Disorder* 207: 188–196.

88. Noorafshan, A., M. Vafabin, S. Karbalay-Doust, and R. Asadi-Golshan. 2017. "Efficacy of curcumin in the modulation of anxiety provoked by sulfite, a food preservative, in rats." *Preventative Nutrition and Food Science* 22 (2): 144–148.

89. Wu, A., E. E. Noble, E. Tyagi, Z. Ying, Y. Zhuang, and F. Gomez-Pinilla. 2015. "Curcumin boosts DHA in the brain: Implications for the prevention of anxiety disorders." *Biochimica et Biophysica Acta* 1852 (5): 951–961.

90. Biswas, J., D. Sinha, S. Mukherjee, S. Roy, M. Siddiqi, and M. Roy. 2010. "Curcumin protects DNA damage in a chronically arsenic-exposed population of West Bengal." *Human and Experimental Toxicology* 29 (6): 513–524.

91. Purohit, R. N., M. Bhatt, K. Purohit, J. Acharya, R. Kumar, and R. Garg. 2017. "Clinical and radiological evaluation of turmeric powder as a pulpotomy medicament in primary teeth: An in vivo study." *International Journal of Clinical Pediatric Dentistry* 10 (1): 37–40.

92. Srivastava, R., V. Puri, R. C. Srimal, and B. N. Dhawan. 1986. "Effect of curcumin on platelet aggregation and vascular prostacyclin synthesis." *Arzneimittelforschung* 36 (4): 715–717.

93. Rainey-Smith, S. R., B. M. Brown, H. R. Sohrabi, T. Shah, K. G. Goozee, V. B. Gupta, and R. N. Martins. 2016. "Curcumin and cognition: a randomised, placebo-controlled, double-blind study of community-dwelling older adults." *British Journal of Nutrition* 115 (12): 2106–2113.

94. Wu, A., E. E. Noble, E. Tyagi, Z. Ying, Y. Zhuang, and F. Gomez-Pinilla. 2015. "Curcumin boosts DHA in the brain: Implications for the prevention of anxiety disorders." *Biochimica Biophysica Acta* 1852 (5): 951–961.

95. Zandi, K., E. Ramedani, K. Mohammadi, S. Tajbakhsh, I. Deilami, Z. Rastian, M. Fouladvand, F. Yousefi, and F. Farshadpour. 2010. "Evaluation of antiviral activities of curcumin derivatives against HSV-1 in Vero cell line." *Natural Product Communications* 5 (12): 1935–1938.

96. Yang, X. X., C. M. Li, and C. Z. Huang. 2016. "Curcumin modified silver nanoparticles for highly efficient inhibition of respiratory syncytial virus infection." *Nanoscale* 8 (5): 3040–3048.

97. Zuccotti, G. V., D. Trabattoni, M. Morelli, S. Borgonovo, L. Schneider, and M. Clerici. 2009. "Immune modulation by lactoferrin and curcumin in children with recurrent respiratory infections." *Journal of Biological Regulators & Homeostatic Agents* 23 (2): 119–123.

98. Xu, Y., B. S. Ku, H. Y. Yao, Y. H. Lin, X. Ma, Y. H. Zhang, and X. J. Li. 2005. "The effects of curcumin on depressive-like behaviors in mice." *European Journal of Pharmacology* 518 (1): 40–46.

99. Lopresti, A. L., and P. D. Drummond. 2017. "Efficacy of curcumin, and a saffron/curcumin combination for the treatment of major depression: A randomised, double-blind, placebo-controlled study." *Journal of Affective Disorders* 207: 188–196.

100. Sanmukhani, J., V. Satodia, J. Trivedi, T. Patel, D. Tiwari, B. Panchal, A. Goel, and C. B. Tripathi. 2014. "Efficacy and safety of curcumin in major depressive disorder: a randomized controlled trial." *Phytotherapy Research* 28 (4): 579–585.

101. Sasidharan, N. K., S. R. Sreekala, J. Jacob, B. Nambisan. 2014. "In vitro synergistic effect of curcumin in combination with third generation cephalosporins against bacteria associated with infectious diarrhea." *Biomedical Research International* 2014: 561456.

102. Chen, M., D. N. Hu, Z. Pan, C. W. Lu, C. Y. Xue, and I. Aass. 2010. "Curcumin protects against hyperosmoticity-induced IL-1beta elevation in human corneal epithelial cell via MAPK pathways." *Experimental Eye Research* 90 (3): 437–443.

103. Trinh, H. T., E. A. Bae, J. J. Lee, and D. H. Kim. 2009. "Inhibitory effects of curcuminoids on passive cutaneous anaphylaxis reaction and scratching behavior in mice." *Archives of Pharmaceutical Research* 32 (12): 1783–1787.

104. Pakfetrat, M., F. Basiri, L. Malekmakan, and J. Roozbeh. 2014. "Effects of turmeric on uremic pruritus in end stage renal disease patients: a double-blind randomized clinical trial." *Journal of Nephrology* 27 (2): 203–207.

105. Lee, H. S., E. J. Choi, K. S. Lee, H. R. Kim, B. R. Na, M. S. Kwon, G. S. Jeong, H. G. Choi, E. Y. Choi, and C. D. Jun. 2016. "Oral administration of p-hydroxycinnamic acid attenuates atopic dermatitis by downregulating Th1 and Th1 cytokine production and keratinocyte activation." *PLoS One* 11 (3): e0150952.

106. Tyagi, P., et al., "Bactericidal activity of curcumin I is associated with damaging of bacterial membrane."

107. Lal, B., A. K. Kapoor, O. P. Asthana, P. K. Agrawal, R. Prasad, P. Kumar, and R. C. Srimal. 1999. "Efficacy of curcumin in the management of chronic anterior uveitis." *Phytotherapy Research* 13 (4): 318–322.

108. Xu, Y., and L. Liu. 2017. "Curcumin alleviates macrophage activation and lung inflammation induced by influenza virus infection through inhibiting the NF-κB signaling pathway." *Influenza and Other Respiratory Viruses* 11 (5): 457–463.

109. Chen, T. Y., D. Y. Chen, H. W. Wen, J. L. Ou, S. S. Chiou, J. M. Chen, M. L. Wong, and W. L. Hsu. 2013. "Inhibition of enveloped viruses infectivity by curcumin." *PLoS One* 8 (5): e62482.

110. Venkatesan, N. 1998. "Curcumin attenuation of acute adriamycin myocardial toxicity in rats." *British Journal of Pharmacology* 124 (3): 425–427.

111. Sannia, A. 2010. "Phytotherapy with a mixture of dry extracts with hepatoprotective effects containing artichoke leaves in the management of functional dyspepsia symptoms." *Minerva Gastroenterologica e Dietologica* 56 (2): 93–99.

112. Thamlikitkul, V., N. Bunyapraphatsara, T. Dechatiwongse, S. Theerapong, C. Chantrakul, T. Thanaveerasuwan, S. Nimitnon, P. Boonroj, W. Punkrut, V. Gingsungneon V, et al. 1989. "Randomized double blind study of *Curcuma domestica* Val. for dyspepsia." *Journal of the Medical Association of Thailand* 72: 613–620.

113. Bundy, R., A. F. Walker, R. W. Middleton, and J. Booth. 2004. "Turmeric extract may improve irritable bowel syndrome symptomology in otherwise healthy adults: a pilot study." *Journal of Alternative and Complementary Medicine* 10 (6): 1015–1018.

114. ScienceDaily. "Method to Prevent Liver Damage Induced by Anti-Tuberculosis Treatment?" *World Journal of Gastroenterology*, September 19, 2008. https://www.sciencedaily.com/releases/2008/09/080919142358.htm.

115. Adhvaryu, M. R., N. Reddy, and B. C. Vakharia. 2008. "Prevention of hepatotoxicity due to anti tuberculosis treatment: a novel integrative approach." *World Journal of Gastroenterology* 14 (30): 4753–4762.

116. Abdel-Daim, M. M., and R. H. Abdou. 2015. "Protective effects of diallyl sulfide and curcumin separately against thallium-induced toxicity in rats." *The Cell Journal* 17: 379–388.

117. Reddy, A.C. and B. R. Lokesh. 1996. "Effect of curcumin and eugenol on iron-induced hepatic toxicity in rats." *Toxicology* 107: 39–45.

118. Rukkumani, R., K. Aruna, P. S. Varma, and V. P. Menon. 2004. "Curcumin influences hepatic expression patterns of matrix metalloproteinases in liver toxicity." *Italian Journal of Biochemistry* 53: 61–66.

119. Abdolahi, M., A. Tafakhori, M. Togha, A. A. Okhovat, F. Siassi, M. R. Eshraghian, M. Sedighiyan, M. Djalali, N. Mohammadzadeh Honarvar, and M. Djalali. 2017. "The synergistic effects of ω-3 fatty acids and nano-curcumin supplementation on tumor necrosis factor (TNF)-α gene expression and serum level in migraine patients." *Immunogenetics* 69 (6): 371–378.

120. Nicol, L. M., D. S. Rowlands, R. Fazakerly, and J. Kellett. 2015. "Curcumin supplementation likely attenuates delayed onset muscle soreness (DOMS)." *European Journal of Applied Physiology* 115 (8): 1769–1777.

121. Sharma S., S. K. Kulkarni, J. N. Agrewala, and K. Chopra. 2006. "Curcumin attenuates thermal hyperalgesia in a diabetic mouse model of neuropathic pain." *European Journal of Pharmacology* 536 (3): 256–261.

122. Srinivasan, "Effect of curcumin on blood sugar as seen in a diabetic subject."

123. Wickenberg, J., S. L. Ingemansson, and J. Hlebowicz. 2010. "Effects of *Curcuma longa* (turmeric) on postprandial plasma glucose and insulin in healthy subjects." *Nutrition Journal* 9: 43.

124. Thomas, A. E., B. Varma, S. Kurup, R. Jose, M. L. Chandy, S. P. Kumar, M. S. Aravind, and A. A. Ramadas. 2017. "Evaluation of efficacy of 1% curcuminoids as local application in management of oral lichen planus—interventional study." *Journal of Clinical Diagnostic Research* 11 (4): ZC89–ZC93.

125. Riva, A., S. Togni, L. Giacomelli, F. Franceschi, R. Eggenhoffner, B. Feragalli, G. Belcaro, M. Cacchio, H. Shu, and M. Dugall. 2017. "Effects of a curcumin-based supplementation in asymptomatic subjects with low bone density: a preliminary 24-week supplement study." *European Review for Medical and Pharmacological Sciences* 21 (7): 1684–1689.

126. Khayat, S., H. Fanaei, M. Kheirkhah, Z. B. Moghadam, A. Kasaeian, and M. Javadimehr. 2015. "Curcumin attenuates severity of premenstrual syndrome symptoms: A randomized, double-blind, placebo-controlled trial." *Complementary Therapies in Medicine* 23 (3): 318–324.

127. Carrion-Gutierrez, M., A. Ramirez-Bosca, V. Navarro-Lopez, A. Martinez-Andres, M. Asín-Llorca, A. Bernd, and J. F. Horga de la Parte. 2015. "Effects of curcuma extract and visible light on adults with plaque psoriasis." *European Journal of Dermatology* 25 (3): 240–246.

128. Bradford, P. G. 2013. "Curcumin and obesity." *Biofactors* 39 (1): 78–87.

129. Di Pierro, F., A. Bressan, D. Ranaldi, G. Rapacioli, L. Giacomelli, and A. Bertuccioli. 2015. "Potential role of bioavailable curcumin in weight loss and omental adipose tissue decrease: preliminary data of a randomized, controlled trial in overweight people with metabolic syndrome. Preliminary study." *European Review for Medical and Pharmacology Sciences* 19 (21): 4195–4202.

130. Teich, T., J. A. Pivovarov, D. P. Porras, E. C. Dunford, and M. C. Riddell. 2017. "Curcumin limits weight gain, adipose tissue growth, and glucose intolerance following the cessation of exercise and caloric restriction in rats." *Journal of Applied Physiology (1985)* 123 (6): 1625–1624.

131. Tawatsin, A., S. D. Wratten, R. R. Scott, U. Thavara, and Y. Techadamrongsin. 2001. "Repellency of volatile oils from plants against three mosquito vectors." *Journal of Vector Ecology* 26: 76–82.

132. Singha, S., and G. Chandra. 2011. "Mosquito larvicidal activity of some common spices and vegetable waste on *Culex quinquefasciatus* and *Anopheles stephensi*." *Asian Pacific Journal of Tropical Medicine* 4 (4): 288–293.

133. Partoazar, A., N. Kianvash, M. H. Darvishi, S. Nasoohi, S. M. Rezayat, and A. Bahador. 2016. "Ethosomal curcumin promoted wound healing and reduced bacterial flora in second degree burn in rat." *Drug Resistance* 66 (12): 660–665.

134. Sidhu, G. S., H. Mani, J. P. Gaddipati, A. K. Singh, P. Seth, K. K. Banaudha, G. K. Patnaik, and R. K. Maheshwari. 1999. "Curcumin enhances wound healing in streptozotocin induced diabetic rats and genetically diabetic mice." *Wound Repair and Regeneration* 7 (5): 362–374.

135. Auysawasdi, N., S. Chuntranuluck, S. Phasomkusolsil, and V. Keeratinijakal. 2016. "Improving the effectiveness of three essential oils against *Aedes aegypti* (Linn.) and *Anopheles dirus* (Peyton and Harrison)." *Parasitology Research* 115 (1): 99–106.

136. Ali, A., Y. H. Wang, and I. A. Khan. 2015. "Larvicidal and biting deterrent activity of essential oils of *Curcuma longa*, ar-turmerone, and curcuminoids against *Aedes aegypti* and *Anopheles quadrimaculatus* (Culicidae: Diptera)." *Journal of Medical Entomology* 52 (5): 979–986.

137. Liu, C. H., and H. Y. Huang. 2013. "In vitro anti-propionibacterium activity by curcumin containing vesicle system." *Chemical and Pharmaceutical Bulletin* (Tokyo) 61 (4): 419–425.

138. Rasheed, A., G. Avinash Kumar Reddy, S. Mohanalakshmi, and C. K. Ashok Kumar. 2011. "Formulation and comparative evaluation of poly herbal anti-acne face wash gels." *Pharmaceutical Biology* 49 (8): 771–774.

139. Tu, C. X., M. Lin, S. S. Lu, X. Y. Qi, R. X. Zhang, and Y. Y. Zhang. 2012. "Curcumin inhibits melanogenesis in human melanocytes." *Phytotherapy Research* 26 (2): 174–179.

140. Agrawal, R., and I. P. Kaur. 2010. "Inhibitory effect of encapsulated curcumin on ultraviolet-induced photoaging in mice." *Rejuvenation Research* 13 (4): 397–410.

141. Sikora, E., G. Scapagnini, and M. Barbagallo. 2010. "Curcumin, inflammation, ageing and age-related diseases." *Immunity & Ageing* 20107: 1.

142. Partoazar, A., et al., "Ethosomal curcumin promoted wound healing and reduced bacterial flora in second degree burn in rat."

143. Heng, M. C. 2013. "Signaling pathways targeted by curcumin in acute and chronic injury: burns and photo-damaged skin." *International Journal of Dermatology* 52 (5): 531–543.

144. Kianvash, N., A. Bahador, M. Pourhajibagher, H. Ghafari, V. Nikoui, S. M. Rezayat, A. R. Dehpour, and A. Partoazar. 2017. "Evaluation of propylene glycol nanoliposomes containing curcumin on burn wound model in rat: biocompatibility, wound healing, and anti-bacterial effects." *Drug Delivery and Translational Research* 7 (5): 642–653.

145. Cheppudira, B., M. Fowler, L. McGhee, A. Greer, A. Mares, L. Petz, D. Devore, D. R. Loyd, and J. L. Clifford. 2013. "Curcumin: a novel therapeutic for burn pain and wound healing." *Expert Opinion on Investigational Drugs* 22 (10): 1295–1303.

146. Partoazar, A., et al., "Ethosomal curcumin promoted wound healing and reduced bacterial flora in second degree burn in rat."

147. Ibid.

148. Pakfetrat, M., F. Basiri, L. Malekmakan, and J. Roozbeh. 2014. "Effects of turmeric on uremic pruritus in end stage renal disease patients: a double-blind randomized clinical trial." *Journal of Nephrology* 27 (2): 203–207.

149. Jia, S., P. Xie, S. J. Hong, R. Galiano, A. Singer, R. A. Clark, and T. A. Mustoe. 2014. "Intravenous curcumin efficacy on healing and scar formation in rabbit ear wounds under nonischemic, ischemic, and ischemia-reperfusion conditions." *Wound Repair and Regeneration* 22 (6): 730–739.

150. Tawatsin, A., et al., "Repellency of volatile oils from plants against three mosquito vectors."

151. Pakfetrat, M., et al., "Effects of turmeric on uremic pruritus in end stage renal disease patients: a double-blind randomized clinical trial."

152. Panahi, Y., A. Sahebkar, M. Amiri, S. M. Davoudi, F. Beiraghdar, S. L. Hoseininejad, and M. Kolivand. 2012. "Improvement of sulphur mustard-induced chronic pruritus, quality of life and antioxidant status by curcumin: results of a randomised, double-blind, placebo-controlled trial." *British Journal of Nutrition* 108 (7): 1272–1279.

153. Trinh, H. T., et al., "Inhibitory effects of curcuminoids on passive cutaneous anaphylaxis reaction and scratching behavior in mice."

154. Srivilai, J., K. Rabgay, N. Khorana, N. Waranuch, N. Nuengchamnong, W. Wisuitiprot, T. Chuprajob, C. Changtam, A. Suksamrarn, W. Chavasiri, N. Sornkaew, and K. Ingkaninan. 2017. "Anti-androgenic curcumin analogues as steroid 5-alpha reductase inhibitors." *Medicinal Chemistry Research* 26 (7): 1550–1556.

155. Zaman, Shahiquz, and Naveed Akhtar. 2013. "Effect of turmeric (*Curcuma longa Zingiberaceae*) extract cream on human skin sebum secretion." *Tropical Journal of Pharmaceutical Research* 12 (5).

156. Asawanonda, P., and S. O. Klahan. 2010. "Tetrahydrocurcuminoid cream plus targeted narrowband UVB phototherapy for vitiligo: a preliminary randomized controlled study." *Photomedicine Laser Surgery* 28 (5): 679–684.

ABOUT THE AUTHOR

SUSAN BRANSON earned an undergraduate degree in biology from St. Francis Xavier University, then an MSc in toxicology from the University of Ottawa. From there, she worked in research: in the field, in the lab, as a writer, and as an administrator. She took time off and stayed at home after her second child was born. In addition to being a stay-at-home mom, she also took violin lessons, took photography courses, earned a diploma in writing, and ultimately became a holistic nutritional consultant. Susan is a member of CSNN's Alumni Association, Canada's leading holistic nutrition school.

ABOUT FAMILIUS

VISIT OUR WEBSITE: WWW.FAMILIUS.COM
JOIN OUR FAMILY

There are lots of ways to connect with us! Subscribe to our newsletters at www.familius.com to receive uplifting daily inspiration, essays from our Pater Familius, a free ebook every month, and the first word on special discounts and Familius news.

GET BULK DISCOUNTS

If you feel a few friends and family might benefit from what you've read, let us know and we'll be happy to provide you with quantity discounts. Simply email us at orders@familius.com.

CONNECT

Facebook: www.facebook.com/paterfamilius
Twitter: @familiustalk, @paterfamilius1
Pinterest: www.pinterest.com/familius
Instagram: @familiustalk

FAMILIUS

THE MOST IMPORTANT WORK YOU EVER DO WILL BE WITHIN THE WALLS OF YOUR OWN HOME.